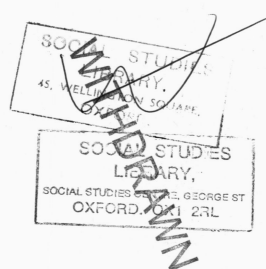

Readings in GERONTOLOGY

READINGS IN GERONTOLOGY

Edited by

VIRGINIA M. BRANTL, Ph.D.

Professor, College of Human Development, and Director of Nursing
and Nursing Education, Milton S. Hershey Medical Center Campus
of the Pennsylvania State University,
Hershey, Pennsylvania

SISTER MARIE RAYMOND BROWN, R.S.M., M.N.Ed.

Formerly Assistant Professor of Nursing, Psychiatric-Mental Health,
School of Nursing, University of Rochester,
Rochester, New York

THE C. V. MOSBY COMPANY

Saint Louis   1973

Printed in the United States of America

Distributed in Great Britain by Henry Kimpton, London

Library of Congress Cataloging in Publication Data

Brantl, Virginia M   1925- comp.
   Readings in gerontology.

   CONTENTS: Maddox, G. L. Themes and issues in
sociological theories of human aging.—Shock, N. W.
Age with a future.—Birren, J. E. Research on aging:
a frontier of science and social gain.—Neugarten,
B. L. Developmental perspectives. [etc.]
    1. Geriatrics—Addresses, essays, lectures.
I. Brown, Marie Raymond, 1931-   joint comp.
II. Title. [DNLM: 1. Geriatrics—Collected works.
WT   100   B821r   1973]
RC952.B7   618.9'7'008   73-90
ISBN   0-8016-0733-7

E/M/M 9 8 7 6 5 4 3 2

FOREWORD

Gerontology, the study of aging, is a relatively new area of scientific inquiry. With increasing numbers of older persons in the population, major issues in regard to our social policies and practices toward the aging have arisen. The phenomenon of aging has had a major impact on our social arrangements and institutions, including the family, government, and the political process and income maintenance and work, as well as in the areas of health and social welfare delivery systems.

The application of knowledge to human aging requires multidisciplinary focus. Thus for those who would develop programs of services or who would prepare persons to work with older people, there is need for an interdisciplinary approach. In addition, there is an interdependence among practice, training, and research. Those who would work with older persons must have, in addition to humanistic values and skills, knowledge of the theories of aging—biological, sociological, and psychological—the relevant research in these areas, and a view as to how such theories and research findings may be applied through practice. There is a further need for training practitioners in needed skills as well as perspectives for a new generation of practitioners in the health, social, and rehabilitative professions. Finally, practitioners must learn to identify and organize the data and social facts that grow out of practice and relate these to the university and research laboratories so that research may raise the right questions and develop new perspectives regarding the social usefulness of such research.

Through the perceptive editorship of Dr. Virginia M. Brantl and Sister Marie Raymond Brown, this set of readings has been organized to provide the reader with an understanding of the relationship between theory, research, and practice. Included are papers presenting some of the "cutting edges" of gerontology. Having these writings organized under one cover should be useful to the practitioner, the teacher, and the student.

There is, indeed, a need to develop commitments to and identities with the aging among the young, the educators, and those seeking middle careers. Due to our cultural and social biases, there is a shortage of curriculum offerings in gerontology in our universities and colleges and vast shortages in trained manpower to work toward meeting the varied needs of our approximately 21 million persons over 65 years of age. This book of readings should help to develop such commitments by pointing the way, through concepts and knowledge of the status of research and some of the major issues in gerontology. Furthermore, it should serve as a bridge between knowledge and practice concerning some of the major issues confronting older persons.

Walter M. Beattie, Jr.
Director, All-University Gerontology Center,
Syracuse University, Syracuse, New York

PREFACE

Older persons in our society have in a sense been pioneers in that advances in technology and health care have enhanced the chances of living to an age that only a few generations ago would have been the exception to the rule. Since the effects of the aging process are not uniform, there also seems to be no way to determine the sequence of study of these phenomena. Hence a continual search for comprehensive theories and their application is vital so that we may understand the complexities of the forces at work in this phase of the life span.

Whereas increasing numbers of monographs, articles, and reading texts have been devoted to the problems of our aging population, numerous other concepts and empirical findings related to the psychological, physiological, and sociological aspects of the lives of our elderly citizens have appeared in a highly fragmented fashion in the literature. Because of the nature of this isolation of the reportable data, for this book we chose to select readings that would tie together underlying concepts and principles directed toward a multidisciplinary approach to the study of the aged. No attempt has been made, however, to cover any of these contributions comprehensively, since in time these selections could be added to or modified as our understanding of the aging process becomes more accurate and predictable.

The aim of this book of readings, therefore, was to select a systematic ordering of the most recent and relevant issues, which, it is hoped, will generate further research and implementation of theories in those disciplines related to the field of gerontology. This volume has the advantage of containing a variety of sources representative of the disciplines of gerontology, psychology, physiology, medical science, sociology, social work, genetics, and nutrition.

We wish to express our sincere gratitude and appreciation to our contributors for granting us permission to reproduce their ideas and suggestions. We wish also to acknowledge the many people who have been of assistance to us in the preparation of this book. Sister Mary Clare Bollow, acting as secretary to the editors, handled all correspondence with the publishers and authors and maintained records. Her assistance was invaluable. Mrs. Lucretia McClure of the Edward G. Miner Library at the University of Rochester Medical Center and Mrs. Ruby Smith, Reference Librarian at the Milton Hershey Medical Center of the Pennsylvania State University, were untiring in their search of the literature and their offers of technical assistance.

Walter M. Beattie, Jr., Director of the All-University Gerontology Center at Syracuse University and formerly Dean of the School of Social Work at Syracuse, kindly agreed to write the foreword for this book. Much of the motivation and momentum for this work was due to the workshops on gerontology that Walter Beattie led during 1970-1972. Mrs. Dorothy Johnson, Project Director for those workshops, was also responsible for initiating our interest in preparing such an anthology.

Virginia M. Brantl
Sister Marie Raymond Brown

CONTENTS

Themes and issues in sociological theories of human aging*

GEORGE L. MADDOX**

Sociological interest in theoretical explanations of human aging has increased markedly in the past three decades. This explicit interest reflects both the increasing social visibility of the old in modern societies and the realization that investigation of older people provides an opportunity to test many basic propositions about the determinants and consequences of social behavior generally.

Social integration of the old

The social visibility of the old has increased dramatically. Technological innovations in the recent past have increased life expectancy and have resulted in the doubling of the proportion of older people in many societies. This visibility of numbers has been accentuated by public discussion of politically feasible programs and adequate services for meeting the needs of the old. The personal troubles of many of the most visible old have come to be perceived cumulatively as a social problem which warrants explanation as well as solution. Initially the problems of the old—medical, economic, and social—which were increasingly acute and clearly warranted attention were more obvious than either solutions or

Reproduced from Human Development 13:17-27, 1970.
*Presented at the First Plenary Session, 8th International Congress of Gerontology, Washington, D.C., August 25, 1969. Preparation of the paper was supported in part by grant HD-668, National Institute of Child Health and Human Development, and by a Special Post-Doctoral Research Fellowship, Center for Health Care Research and Development, U.S.P.H.S.
**Department of Psychiatry and Sociology, Duke University, Durham, North Carolina.

explanations. But plausible explanations were available, particularly from sociological theorists who were already concerned about the viability of institutional arrangements in urban, industrial societies generally. In such societies all existing values and social arrangements were considered to be vulnerable and change was believed to be epidemic. Every individual was perceived to be vulnerable, the old particularly so.

The explanation of the problematic aspects of living in modern urban societies, which was initially and repeatedly advanced, thus focused on their institutional arrangements. These were said to be especially uncongenial to the needs of the old and to their integration into the mainstream of social life. Sociologists interested in the family feared that the centrality of the small, isolated, conjugal family unit and geographic mobility inevitably led to the isolation of the old from kinsmen. Industrial sociologists viewed with alarm the high probability of technological obsolescence among all workers and substantial increases in nonwork time for which few were prepared; the old seemed especially vulnerable. Students of culture were sadly convinced that, in societies bound to the wheel of rapid change, youth would be valued and the old depreciated. In sum, the problems of the old appeared to flow predictably and inexorably from the uncongenial institutional arrangements of modern societies.

The initial evidence seemed to support this pessimistic theorizing. In the United States as elsewhere, for example, early characterizations of the old depicted them as socially isolated, impoverished, disabled, and psychologically alienated. Although the prognosis for the social integration of the old seemed poor, the prevailing humane prescription called for the amelioration of their unfortunate circumstances as much as possible within the existing institutional arrangements. Liberalized social welfare arrangements and intensified social work seemed indicated to minimize the impoverishment and social isolation of the old.

The conclusion that urban, industrial societies are institutionally uncongenial to the old seemed plausible enough. But there were some investigators who were unconvinced. In the first place, some skeptical research investigators noted that the dominant characterizations of the old were frequently based on visible but unrepresentative samples of the institutionalized old or of those older persons in contact with welfare agencies. Moreover, there were others who considered the idyllic descriptions of the social integration of the old in preindustrial societies as somewhat romanticized. What were the facts?

The facts were that careful studies of older people living normally in communities, where most older people actually live, failed to validate the gloomy expectations predicted by prevailing theory and inadequate research. The old simply cannot be accurately described as usually disabled from illness, economically destitute, or psychologically alienated. On the contrary most older people in urban, industrial societies, believed to be the most uncongenial to the elderly, have been found to be reasonably competent in meeting their needs socially as well as personally. Moreover, recent cross-national research has provided a crucial test of the theory that urban, industrial societies preclude the integration of the old, and has rejected it. Investigators in the United States, in England, and in Denmark have used probability samples of old people to produce definitive evidence on this point.[1, 2, 3] The more optimistic current estimates of the possibility of integrating older people in contemporary society do not require that one ignore the substantial minority of the old for whom personal and social problems persist, often in acute form. But the evidence no longer permits the conclusions that aging in contemporary society precludes satisfactory integration and adaptation of the old, that satisfactory integration and adaptation are the experience of a minority only, or that in less complex types of societies growing old is unproblematic. Furthermore, the need for greater specificity in describing and explaining problems of aging and of the aged has been repeatedly demonstrated. For instance, older persons are overrepresented among persons with income below the poverty level in the United States. Being older, and by implication more likely to be unemployed or retired, clearly is associated with economic poverty for a substantial minority. But it is equally important to stress that, while too many older persons may be impoverished, most are not. Even among those who are impoverished a large though undertermined proportion have a history of economic marginality throughout their adult years, not just in the later years. Similarly, retirement from work for males and the loss of contact with children for females have frequently been described as the inevitable traumatic experiences of the later years. The assumption of trauma associated with these common experiences simply does not square with the facts. Retirement from work and changing relationships with children take many forms and have different meanings; it has not been demonstrated that *traumatic* is an accurate description of the most probable response to these experiences by most older persons.[4]

Successful aging

As the essential social integration of the old in modern societies was being convincingly demonstrated, a new theoretical issue emerged which was to become the theoretical preoccupation of the decade. The issue was 'successful aging.' The controversial formula for achieving this desired state of affairs was disengagement theory.[5] Cumming and Henry and other disengagement theorists did not focus primarily on the social integration of the old, nor did they quarrel with the conclusion that older people were or could be socially integrated to a satisfactory degree. Rather they contested the assumption that older people must be fully integrated socially, for as long as possible, in the interest of maintaining a satisfactory sense of well-being. On theoretical grounds this was considered to be bad advice. Such advice, they felt, was based on a misunderstanding of the apparent tendency of society and older people to withdraw from each other. Even under optimal personal and social circumstances, the disengagement theorists argued, decreased physical and psychic energy characterize the later years of the life cycle. The result is decreasing social involvement and activity; and equally important, ego involvement in external objects and events decreases. These changes in individuals are part of the ground plan of human organisms. Since the underlying factors are fundamentally intrinsic, the process of withdrawal is inevitable. Moreover, and this was the important point, the mutual withdrawal of society and individual from each other constitutes a necessary condition of successful aging and societal functioning. Evidence was presented in support of this conclusion.

The impact of this sophisticated, tightly-argued interpretation of human aging has been enormous, and the debate it has generated has been very productive. In the balance, disengagement theory has been found wanting empirically and its original formulation is rarely defended by anyone, including its original proponents.[6-11] But there is no question that theoretical understanding of aging as a process has been advanced as has our understanding of the multiple 'successful' variants of this process. We are now reasonably confident, for example, that for most older people the maintenance of a relatively high level of social involvement and activity contributes significantly to a sense of well-being. This remains so even though the level of involvement and activity does characteristically diminish with age. At the same time, we have a new appreciation of the variety of life styles which appear to be 'successful,' that is, which appear to reflect satisfactory articulation of personal needs with social expectations. Although the motivation to conform socially does appear to weaken in the later years, competent social behavior in a variety of forms nevertheless appears to be the rule among the old.

The study of process

Of equal importance, the debate over disengagement theory has raised important methodological issues.[11-16] It is now generally conceded that crucial research on aging as a process must eventually include longitudinal observations or an adequate approximation of such observations. Conventional cross-sectional survey research provides an inadequate basis for the study of developmental processes in general and specifically for partialing out the effects of age changes and of age differences which reflect the varying experiences and socio-cultural environments of successive cohorts. Research experience suggests that the demographic characteristics, social competence, behavior, and attitudes of a given cohort of persons seventy-five years of age, for example, provide a questionable basis for predicting the state of affairs for a cohort of persons sixty-five years of age when they are ten years older. If human aging is in fact as complex a bio-social process as research suggests that it is, then the methodology of research which is appropriate for disentangling the interaction and contribution of biological, psychological and situational factors in this complex process must be much more sophisticated than has typically been the case in social gerontological research in previous decades. Fortunately evidence of the *END* requisite sophistication is increasingly found in the literature.

In the recent past, then, two important theoretical issues in social gerontology have been posed and resolved in a convincing fashion. Important methodological issues have also been clarified. The institutional structure of urban, industrial society is viable for the old. And, within that structure, competent social interaction is not only the rule, it also makes an important contribution to the sense of well-being among the old. Sociological theorists are now turning their attention increasingly to the elaboration and specification of the implications of these conclusions.

The current status of social gerontological theory

A review of the current status of sociological theory in regard to human aging indicated some important and promising developments. The confirmation status of theory in social gerontology is improving. The logical structure of its propositions and arguments is being elaborated in a cumulative fashion. The determinancy of predictions based on theory has increased. The scope of theory in social gerontology is expanding. These encouraging signs of vitality in social gerontological theory warrant brief elaboration.

The confirmation status of theory in social gerontology is improving. Theoretically derived propositions have been and are being posed and decisively tested. Modified extended kinship structure demonstrably continues to exist in complex societies, for example. The density of age-peers of similar social status is positively associated with the amount of social interaction which old people display. Social activity is a positive correlate of a sense of well-being. These propositions only hint at the extensive and expanding catalogue of hypotheses about various aspects of human aging as a social process which are testable and, in many instances, have been already adequately tested. Stereotypic, untested propositions about aging as a social process continue to be generated. An enormous amount of professional energy has been and is still being devoted to disposing of plausible but gratuitous assumptions about growing old. This must be done in the interest of moving toward a theoretically adequate conceptual framework for studying processes of aging. Much obviously remains to be done. Current sociological research in gerontology, however, clearly demonstrates a new interest in the vital interaction of theory and research, which is bringing theoretical and methodological issues more sharply into focus. Stereotypes of the aged and assumptions about aging as a social process increasingly evoke appropriate evidence, and evoke it more quickly than in the past. The life expectancy of gratuitous assumptions is decreasing. The productive controversies about the viability of contemporary institutional arrangements for the old, and about the distribution and consequences of social involvement of the old illustrate the point. Sources of information about aging and the aged are increasingly more common, more reliable, more available and, consequently, more frequently consulted and appropriately used.

The logical structure of theory in social gerontology is being elaborated and specified in a cumulative fashion. Extensive systematic reviews of the confirmation status of a wide range of propositions and theoretical perspectives in social gerontology have recently been published.[10, 16, 17] It is no longer defensible, for example, and certainly no longer theoretically profitable, to make generalizations about *the aged* as if they constituted a homogeneous category. Age *per se* masks considerable variation in self-conceptions, in the personal and social resources which demonstrably exist among persons of the same chronological age, and in behavior. It is increasingly apparent that theorists must be prepared to specify differences in the content of personal goals and the degree of their achievement if differences in behavior among the old are to be explained. Controls must always be introduced for social status (a variable known to summarize previous life experience), expectations, and opportunities, as well as current resources and goals. Feelings of loneliness can no longer be treated as the inevitable or even probable consequences of social separation among the old. Current specification and elaboration of hypotheses about social aspects of aging reflect awareness shared by social scientists generally that multivariate analysis is as necessary as it is useful in the analysis of complex social processes. Moreover, increasing attention is being given to the methodological problems involved in the diachronic analysis of social phenomena. Understanding the complex interaction of variables and feedback effects in the operation of social and social psychological processes is central to adequate theorizing about aging as well as other phenomena of interest to sociologists. The problems involved in the study of social processes are being identified and addressed with increasing clarity.[12, 13, 18, 19]

The determinacy of predictions based on theory in social gerontology has increased. This follows from the improved confirmation status of theory generally, as noted previously, and from the increased specificity and testability of derived propositions. Social competence, adaptive flexibility, and a sense of well-being displayed by persons in the middle years of life predict the probable display of these same characteristics in the later years. The life cycle may be conceptualized as a process in which success predicts success. The exact combination of personal and social factors which predict successful aging cannot currently be specified. Nor can the primacy of one or another variable in determining successful outcome be determined exactly. This may be so, in part, because different cultures, and subcultures within a single society, propose different standards by which 'success' in aging is evaluated.[20] But more than this, both the social self and society are open systems capable, in interaction, of generating a number of alternative life styles, the outcomes of which are equally satisfactory. Some apparently different, complex bio-social structures and processes seem to have, following the argument of L. Bertalannfy, equipotential for producing adequate outcomes; in this sense the outcomes are equifinal.[21] Moreover, when complex structures and processes are involved, the possibility for morphogenesis must be considered. That is, observed adequate outcomes of processes cannot simply be assumed to exhaust the possibilities.[22] Such considerations lead to the conclusion that no single formula for optimal aging is known or is likely to be found. Most important, on theoretical grounds one might not even expect to find a single solution.

The scope of theory in social gerontology is expanding. Vital linkages with sociological and social psychological theory are evident in a number of areas. Cases in point include theories of kinship structure in modern societies; crisis theory; role theory; theories of socialization and development over the life cycle; theories of social process and change.[3, 22, 23, 24, 25] The development of theory in social gerontology parallels the experience in many substantive areas which are initially occasioned and stimulated by a specific set of problems. Earlier narrow preoccupation with aging *per se* and its problems and the professional isolation of social gerontologists interacting primarily among themselves have increasingly given way to an appreciation of aging as a phenomenon of general sociological relevance and to the integration of social gerontology into the mainstream of sociology. This integration is most pronounced among sociologists with interests in socialization, social integration, social competence, and the comparative analysis of social structure and social change. The relevance of understanding the determinants and consequences of behavior in the middle years of life for understanding the later years of life is being discovered. There is a new interest in sociological aspects of life cycle events and their interrelationships to challenge the earlier provincial preoccupations of investigators with childhood, or adolescence, or old age. The articulation of social gerontological theory and research with policy formation is improving. The disutility of attempting to develop programs for *the* elderly is now clear. Not all elderly persons have the same needs, nor do they require the same services. Future public policy formation will surely reflect this awareness. Moreover, problems associated with growing old are more and more clearly perceived as a barometer indicating problem areas of general significance for society. The old, in a sense, have been pioneers. Their specific problems in adapting to increased leisure have called attention to the general societal relevance of this issue. Similarly, attempts to deal with the medical and welfare problems of the old have stimulated interest in alternative ways in which these problems can be met. These experiences have produced models for delivering care which may be generally applicable to persons of any age. Research on aging has also demonstrated the importance of longitudinal multivariate analysis in the study of social processes and social change and has provided an opportunity to illustrate the relevance of socio-cultural environment in understanding human behavior.

The increasing potential and vitality of sociological theory in gerontology are evident. Cross-national and cross-cultural research will become more common, adding an important dimension to the status of theory in social gerontology. The cross-national research which has already been reported or which will be reported soon has made a significant contribution to comparative sociology. Definitive comparative research on societies significantly different in culture and social structure remains to be done and faces substantial methodological barriers. But such research is possible and becomes more likely as sustained professional interaction of sociologists throughout the world increases. At the same time, there is a new appreciation among sociologists that important variations remain to be explored in aging as a social process within given societies; and it is likely that limited resources will be, and perhaps should be, placed here rather than in cross-cultural research.

In conclusion, then, social gerontological theory is not all that it should be. It is not even all that it might be. But it is considerably more adequate now than it was even one decade ago in its explanation of the social aspects of human aging. The foundation has been laid for more adequate theory and research in the future and social gerontology is finding its place in relation to the established social scientific disciplines.

REFERENCES

1. Shanas, E.; Townsend, P.; Wedderburn, D.; Friis, H.; Milhoj, P. and Strehouwer, J.: Older people in three industrial societies (Atherton Press, New York/London 1968).
2. Shanas, E. and Streib, G. (eds.): Social structure and the family: Generational relations (Prentice-Hall, Englewood Cliffs 1965).
3. Rosenmayr, L.: Family relations of the elderly. J. Marriage Family 30:672-680 (1968).
4. Maddox, G.: Retirement as a social event in the United States; in McKinney and de Vyver, Aging and social policy (Appleton-Century-Crofts, New York 1966).
5. Cumming, E. and Henry, W.: Growing old: The process of disengagement (Basic Books, New York 1961).
6. Cumming, E.: Further thoughts on the theory of disengagement. UNESCO Int. Social Sci. Bull. 15:377-393 (1963).
7. Henry, W.: The theory of intrinsic disengagement; paper presented at the International Gerontological Research Seminar, Markaryd, Sweden, 1963.
8. Rose, A.: A current theoretical issue in social gerontology. Gerontologist 4:46-50 (1964).
9. Maddox, G.: Disengagement theory: A critical evaluation. Gerontologist 4:80-83 (1964).
10. Havighurst, R.; Neugarten, B. and Tobin, S.: Disengagement and patterns of aging; in Neugarten, Middle age and aging (University of Chicago Press, Chicago 1968).
11. Maddox, G.: Fact and artifact: Evidence bearing on disengagement theory from the Duke Geriatric Project. Hum. Develop. 8: (1965).
12. Schaie, W.: A general model for the study of developmental problems. Psychol. Bull. 64:92-107 (1965).
13. Schaie, W.: Age changes and age difference; in Neugarten, Middle age and aging, Appendix C (University of Chicago Press, Chicago 1968).
14. Kagan, C. and Moss, H.: Birth to maturity (Wiley, New York 1962).
15. Ryder, N.: The cohort as a concept in the study of social change. Am. Sociol. Rev. 30:843-861 (1965).

16. Baltes, P. B.: Longitudinal and cross-sectional sequences in the study of age and generation effects. Hum. Develop. 11:145-171 (1968).
17. Riley, M. and Foner, A.: Aging and society: I. An inventory of research findings (Russell Sage Foundation, New York 1968).
18. Rosow, I.: Social integration of the aged (Free Press, New York 1967).
19. Coleman, J.: The mathematical study of change; in Blalock and Blalock, Methodology in social research (McGraw-Hill, New York 1968).
20. Bengston, V.: Cultural and occupational differences in social participation and psychological well-being among retired males: A cross-national study. Unpublished Ph.D Dissertation, University of Chicago (1967).
21. Bertalannfy, L.: Problems of life (Watts, London 1952).
22. Buckley, W.: Sociology and modern systems theory (Prentice-Hall, New York 1967).
23. Clausen, J. (ed.): Socialization and society (Little, Brown, & Co., Boston 1968).
24. Rosow, I.: Socialization to old age; paper presented to a National Institute of Child Health and Human Development Conference on Adult Socialization, San Francisco, CA, 1968.
25. Turner, R.: Role taking: Process or conformity; in Rose, Human behavior and social processes (Houghton Mifflin, New York 1962).

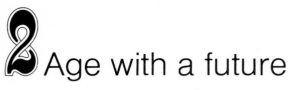

Age with a future

NATHAN W. SHOCK, Ph.D.*

"Father Time is not always a hard parent, and, though he tarries for none of his children, often lays his hand lightly on those who have used him well"—Charles Dickens in "Barnaby Rudge."

The title of this paper is intentionally ambiguous. From it none of you can know whether I plan to write about babies or senescents, since both age. Actually, what I propose to discuss is the total life-span but with special emphasis on the later years.

As indicated, aging is a general universal process which takes place over the entire life-span. The life-span of the human may be roughly divided into three major divisions. During the first 20 years, or even 25 years, of existence, the individual is maturing or learning, but he is also aging. The next 40 years constitute the normal working life. The third period, which may be characterized as the post-retirement period, extends now, for the most part, simply by administrative fiat, from age 65 onward. On the average, this amounts to an additional ten years of life for men and about 17 years for women. These figures represent the best estimates for continued life in individuals who have reached the age of 65. In this paper I would like to explore the potentialities of the post-retirement period and to consider the prospects for improving and extending this period of life.

It must be recognized that the age of retirement is very arbitrary and one which has been fixed in our society as age 65. When the age of 65 was chosen, it was expected that most individuals would spend only about five years in retirement. Now, however, it is apparent that most of us will spend considerably more than five years in retirement. Retirement in the future will be even longer

---

Reproduced from The Gerontologist 8:147-152, Autumn, 1968.
*Gerontology Research Center, National Institute of Child Health and Human Development, National Institutes of Health, PHS, U.S. Department of Health, Education & Welfare, Bethesda, and the Baltimore City Hospitals, Baltimore, Maryland.

since it will begin earlier and last longer. Current trends in technology lead to the prediction that within the foreseeable future the age of retirement for many workers will be lowered to 55.

It is also probable that with advances in medical science there will be a further extension of life-span of as much as five to ten years. Thus, it is increasingly clear that the post-retirement period will encompass a greater proportion of the life-span than it now does and may well represent the period of life when people can reach their ultimate goals of personal achievement and satisfaction. The burning question is, "What do we propose to do with these added years?" *END*.

What are the factors that set a limit on longevity? It is well known that different animals differ widely in their life-span; thus the house fly lives about 90 days, the rat two to three years, the dog 12 to 15, the horse 15 to 20, and man 90 to 100. It is, therefore, clear that the genetic makeup includes some program for aging. Differences in this program, or rate of aging, are present even between individuals within a given species. For example, it has been possible to produce two separate strains of mice, one of which lives only about 12 months whereas the other lives 24 months. Even in man it has been shown that individuals with long lived ancestors live on the average four or five years longer than individuals whose parents and grandparents died at an early age. However, basic biological research has been able to show that whatever this basic genetic pattern of aging is, it can be altered by environmental factors.

In order to conduct experiments of this kind, the investigator must turn to some species other than man. In our laboratory, Dr. Barrows and his associates have studied the effect of changes in temperature and in nutrition on the life-span of the rotifer. The rotifer is a small aquatic animal about the size of a pinhead. It is an ideal animal for these experiments because many individuals can be hatched from eggs laid by the same mother. Since no father is required for this animal, each of the individuals derived from the same mother will have exactly the same genetic program. Since the animal is cold blooded it is also possible to alter its body temperature simply by altering the temperature of the water in which it lives.

Now under normal circumstances this animal has a life-span of approximately 34 days, distributed as follows: four days of development after hatching, 11 to 15 days of active egg laying, and approximately 18 days of "retirement." When the temperature of the animal is raised slightly, that is, from $25°$ to $35°$C. its life-span drops to about 18 days but all of the loss in total life-span comes out of the "retirement" period.

In contrast, life-span can be increased from the normal 34 days to as much as 55 days simply by reducing the food supply available to the animal. However, this alteration in environment does not affect the "retirement" period of life which remains at 18 days. Instead, starvation lengthens life-span by increasing the period of egg-laying from 11 to 29 days, although the total number of eggs laid is the same as in well fed rotifers—it simply takes longer to produce them. The same genetic program for the rotifer can be lengthened or shortened by changes in environmental conditions.

These experimental conditions cannot be applied to the human but they are of extreme importance in showing that the genetic pattern of aging can be influenced by environmental factors. As the biologist generates more basic knowledge about the mechanisms of aging, applications which will benefit people will eventually evolve.

The second most important factor that influences the life-span of the human is disease, of which heart disease, high blood pressure, cancer, and respiratory diseases such as pneumonia are the primary culprits. Arthritis is another common disease; however, it does not kill but produces disability, especially among the elderly.

A third factor which limits longevity is obesity. This is a persistent remedial problem especially among the middle aged.

A fourth factor which limits longevity is the gradual change in organs and tissues which results in a reduction of reserve capacity. These changes do not proceed uniformly in all organ systems and may or may not be the inevitable consequences of aging. It is in this area that a great deal of research needs to be done. We do know that many of these changes can be compensated for by prosthetic devices such as glasses, hearing aids, dentures, etc., and that others can be retarded in their progression by systematic exercise and activities. Others can be lived with simply by avoiding the strain of excesses. A bright future for the aged will stem from (a) contributions of research, (b) the application of medical advances which in turn will be the outgrowth of basic scientific research, (c) the effects of social changes, and (d) the enlightened efforts of the individual himself.

Contribution of research

The problems of aging have been systematically studied only in the past few years. There is a rising interest in studies on the causes of aging at the biological and cellular level but much remains to be done. Few investigators even now are directly concerned with these fundamental problems. In recognition of the need for more investigators in the field of aging, the National Institutes of Health are now supporting some 22 training programs in various aspects of gerontology which have been established in different universities in the United States. Many of these programs are just getting under way and it will be three to five years before a significant number of trained investigators becomes available. However, it is a hopeful sign and a move in the right direction.

Recently a panel of experts of the Rand Corporation has estimated anticipated breakthroughs in various aspects of technology and science. One of their predictions is that by the year 2025 the chemical control of aging will be possible. According to their estimates, artificial organs made of plastic and electronic components will be available by 1990. Biochemicals to stimulate growth of new organs and limbs are predicted by 2020. All of these predictions may sound like science fiction, but who could have predicted 50 years ago that satellites could be put into orbit and a "soft" landing could be made on a pre-selected spot on the moon?

A great deal of research is now being directed toward the underlying causes of many diseases such as heart disease, hardening of the arteries, high blood pressure, cancer, etc. From such research many new drugs for the treatment of high blood pressure and heart disease have been developed. New enzymes have been found which will dissolve blood clots, and intensive efforts are being made to adapt them for use in the human.

One of the important problems for the future is the training of physicians in the special problems of older people. Whether this will be called training in geriatrics or internal medicine is of little consequence. The important issue is that departments of medicine in all medical schools need to develop an awareness among young physicians of the physiological characteristics of older people which are important in treating their ailments and diseases.

Perhaps the most spectacular medical advances have occured in surgery. Artificial tubing can now be substituted for blood vessels which have become blocked. By restoring the blood supply with such artificial blood vessels, many arms and legs which previously had to be amputated can now be saved. Restoring an adequate blood supply to the head with an artificial blood vessel has produced truly remarkable recovery from the effects of stroke in some patients. This technique will undoubtedly be further explored and extended.

I cannot refrain from pointing out that these benefits to patients stemmed from the results of basic research in organic chemistry which made possible the production of plastic and nylon tubes which can be transplanted into the body and do not cause blood to clot. These artificial materials were developed by organic chemists who were originally interested in the chemistry of polymer formation rather than the production of a piece of tubing which could be used inside the body to transport blood.

The development of new synthetic materials has also made possible the construction of artificial valves which can now be transplanted into the human heart to replace leaky ones. Engineering developments such as miniature circuits and batteries have permitted the development of an artificial device known as a "pacemaker" which maintains the heart beat at a regular rate in a patient whose heart misses beats.

A dramatic goal of modern surgery is the transplantation of tissues and organs from one human being to another and ultimately perhaps from animals to man. Transplantation of the kidney, liver, lung, heart, and skin as well as the hormone secreting glands represent ultimate goals. The obstacles that stood in the way of achieving this ambition were surgical, immunological, logistic, and moral. Transplantation of skin from one part of the body to another part in the same person has been possible for a long time, largely because the rejection of the skin by immunological reactions is not a major problem. The grafted skin is recognized by the body as part of itself.

Kidney grafts are also feasible where the donor is a close blood relative of the recipient. Rejection reactions are much less severe toward tissues from close relatives who are apt to be more similar genetically than are people in general. Some of these kidney grafts have remained viable for as long as two to three years. As evidenced by the recent transplantations of human hearts at least the surgical aspects of the problem have been resolved. It is still a moot question as to whether the immunological problems have as yet been solved. The problem is to suppress the immunological responses of the body which reject the grafted organ as a foreign body. Although there are now drugs and methods to accomplish this goal, they are not specific so that the patient loses his ability to fight off any infection. Within the next few years drugs or techniques will probably be developed which will suppress immunologic reaction to heart or kidney tissue but leave intact the ability of the body to produce antibodies against infections.

The logistic problem is one of finding and matching an appropriate donor for each recipient, since we are still a long way from being able to maintain organ banks, although some progress is being made.

At the present time, kidney transplantations are made from living relatives to the patient. This system is possible, since each of us has two kidneys and we can get along pretty well with only one. However, for single organs like the heart, transplants must be made within a short time of the death of the donor. Securing appropriate donors will remain a persistent problem even after all the technical problems are solved.

In my opinion the best escape from the problem of securing donor hearts lies in the development of an artificial pump which can replace the human heart. In the United States a great deal of emphasis is being given to the development of such a device. Engineers, biologists, and physicians are working collaboratively in order to solve the many problems involved. There is, however, no reason a solution, at least for an artificial heart, should not be forthcoming within the foreseeable future.

With the transplantation of other organs the current research approach is to develop techniques whereby organs such as kidney or liver of lower animals can be transplanted to the human. The biological and physiological problems involved in the production of an artificial kidney are much more difficult than for the artificial heart so that the solution is undoubtedly much farther in the future.

The moral problems involved in the transplantation of organs from one human to another are only now becoming apparent. How far are we justified in lowering a donor's expectation of life to prolong the recipient's? What kinds of controls would be required to prevent exploitation of some individuals to provide a source of organs appropriate for transplantation? With the development of artificial organs such as artificial hearts, what limit should be set upon the prolongation of life by these devices? How long should a vegetable existence be extended by artificial means? These are all questions which must be faced by all of us and not just by physicians. Fortunately, we will not be faced with this problem on a mass basis suddenly. It will develop slowly and gradually.

Impending social changes will also play a role in extending the post-retirement period and improving its quality. As previously pointed out, technological advances will undoubtedly tend to lower the age of compulsory retirement. At the same time we can expect a reduction in the length of the work week. This means that during the period of working life more leisure time will become available. With the development of nonworking outside activities, the transition from work to retirement will become less abrupt and, therefore, less traumatic.

With more time available, the worker can engage in many pursuits which can be expanded when he reaches retirement. The middle-aged worker will have more time for community, recreational, and cultural activities than he does at present. He can prepare himself for a second career. A second career does not imply paid employment. A second career may be any activity that is significant and satisfying to the individual. It may range from participation in volunteer community services to fishing, bird watching, or stamp collecting. Its essential characteristic is satisfaction to the individual.

The increasing number of elderly people and lengthening of the post-retirement period demand a redefinition of the role of the elderly. Elderly people must not be regarded simply as a group for whom special services must be provided. Instead they must be regarded as participants in community life. The Age and Opportunity Bureau and other similar organizations must lead the way in demonstrating opportunities for significant roles for the aged within the community.

Senior Centers play an important role in developing social contacts. They have also served as a focal point for cultural and recreational activities. Since only about 5% of the retired population now participate in Senior Center activities, it is apparent that many more are needed and new methods are needed to attract more participants. One approach is to expand programs to channel the efforts of elderly people into useful and significant community activities. This will require not only changes in social customs but also changes in the attitudes of older people. Older individuals, especially men, must be convinced that a pay check is not the only criterion of significant work and efforts. Traditionally, voluntary work within the community is regarded as quite respectable for women but not necessarily for men. This attitude is one which must be overcome if we are to provide meaningful activities for older people.

Ten years ago it was generally assumed that retirement was looked upon as a threat by many people. It was only after research studies directed by Dr. Havighurst and his colleagues in Kansas City that it became apparent that this desire for continued employment was primarily a reflection of the attitudes of professional people and that many older workers looked forward to an actually enjoyed retirement. Hence, the assumption that *all* older people wish to continue to work is wrong. At present over half of the individuals who apply for Social Security benefits in the United States are less than 65 years of age. This is true in spite of the fact that those who retire at age 62 get only 80% of the monthly benefits they would get if they waited until they were 65. It is suggested that one of the reasons so many people are choosing to retire at 62 is that employment opportunities for them have fallen off sharply, in an age stressing automation. Nevertheless, it is apparent that retirement is becoming an acceptable way of life for an increasing proportion of the population.

Social changes will also improve pension benefits. These improvements will accrue not only from increases in benefits such as those enacted by the last Congress of the United States but also from maturation of the retirement program itself. More people will have accumulated increased credits by virtue of longer participation in the program and, therefore, will receive higher retirement incomes.

There should also be marked reduction in the anxiety of aging people with respect to costs for hospitalization and medical care. The enactment of the Medicare program in the United States has provided a firm bases for these services for all people over the age of 65. This program should also improve the health of older people by making available medical services for the treatment of diseases and impairments before they become acute critical problems. It is, therefore, apparent that resources will be available for improving the health status of the elderly. The effectiveness of such programs will depend heavily upon providing physicians, hospitals, and nursing homes as recommended by Dr. Sherman and his committee in a recent report.

Other social programs which will improve the quality of living for elderly people include the development of housing facilities. For the more affluent elderly people, private housing projects and apartment blocks are springing up in many areas of the United States. For those with limited incomes, the requirement established in some states, such as New York, that a certain percentage of the units in public housing projects be allocated to the use of elderly people is a step in the right direction. Federal assistance to non-profit organizations prepared to sponsor construction of new apartments for the elderly has served to stimulate construction of additional units. This trend will continue over the coming years so that improved housing will become more generally available.

There will also be an extension and improvement in services for older people. Homemaker services, day centers, meals on wheels, counseling services, and activity centers will be provided in more and more places through the activities of various agencies. One area which needs extensive exploration is the extent to which elderly people themselves can, through their volunteer activities, provide such services. All of these social changes will contribute greatly to the quality of living in the post-retirement years.

Although research and advances in medical sciences and cultural changes will contribute a great deal to the opportunities of older people for the significant use of their post-retirement years, there are a good many things that the individual himself must do to get the most out of his retirement years. The aging individual must recognize the opportunities that lie before him. First and foremost is the opportunity to be one's self. Freed from economic and social demands of rearing a family, the individual now has the opportunity to choose his own activities and to set his own time schedules. The important point is that, whereas during working life many of his goals have been set by the demands of employment, family, and the need for progressive achievement, the individual now must set his own goals. His goals must be both immediate and long term. It seems to me that perhaps one of the best estimates of the age of an individual would be to inquire about his future plans. As long as the individual has long-term plans he is not really old. He is only old when he has lost all incentive to make plans for his future.

Individuals can also increase their probability of enjoying a long and healthy life by paying closer attention to the quantity and quality of their diet. On the quantitative side, food intake should be adjusted to avoid the accumulation of fat. Insurance statistics show clearly that obesity is associated with an increase in cardiovascular disease and a reduction in life-span.

In a recent study conducted by Dr. Solomon 107 obese men (aged 25-35) who were otherwise normal had decreased biological function tests similar to those of chronologically older men. The greater the obesity, the greater was the impairment. Fifty per cent overweight in a 25-year-old man was associated with functions of heart, lung and kidney and exercise performance found in normal men aged 50. Fifty-two of the originally obese patients reduced to and maintained their ideal weights for one year. At this time, their test results corresponded to those of their chronological age group (25 years). The other 55 patients who remained obese showed no change in their biological tests when repeated a year later.

Although a program of weight reduction will have some beneficial effect, the scars of obesity will remain in the form of sagging skin where the fat came off. This is because one of the basic characteristics of aging is a gradual loss in the elasticity not only of skin but also of blood vessels and other tissues. The old skin is unable to snap back and adjust itself to the new volume once it has been stretched out of shape by the accumulation of fat. Although biologists are engaged in research which may ultimately lead to the development of drugs which can restore the elastic properties to tissues, this goal may be a long way off. It is much better to *keep* slim than to *get* slim.

Since hardening of the arteries is a disease which afflicts a large proportion of elderly people to various degrees and is responsible for heart attacks and strokes, everyone is interested in any method which will prevent the disease or slow it down.

It is now commonly believed that a reduction in fat intake or a shift from the consumption of animal (saturated) fat to vegetable oils (unsaturated) fats will do this. The thesis is that (1) coronary artery disease is associated with high levels of cholesterol and fats in the blood, (2) the level of fats in the blood can be lowered by reducing fat intake and by substituting vegetable oils for animal fat, and (3) lowering the levels of fat and cholesterol in the blood will slow down the rate of development of arteriosclerosis.

The difficulty is that there are still some uncertainties with regard to each of these assumptions that must be resolved by further research. In 1961 the Central Committee for Medical and Community programs of the American Heart Association issued a report on the best scientific information available. It states "reduction of control of fat consumption under medical supervision with reasonable substitution of poly-unsaturated fats is recommended as a possible means in preventing atherosclerosis and decreasing the risk of heart attacks and strokes. . . . more complete information must be obtained before final conclusions can be reached." In 1968 the situation remains essentially the same, although large scale studies are now in progress to test the effects of reduction of fat in the diet on the incidence of arteriosclerosis in well controlled populations.

The studies are extremely difficult to carry out and require a long time before definitive results can be obtained. In the meantime we are again faced with basing action on statistical probabilities. At the present time, a reasonable reduction in the intake of fat, especially animal fat, is probably of benefit to (1) the overweight, (2) those who have already had a heart attack or stroke, and (3) those whose personal family histories suggest that they might be particularly susceptible to arteriosclerosis. There is certainly no final proof as yet that dietary changes can prevent heart attacks or strokes in specific individuals.

The qualitative aspects of diet are also important in health maintenance. Although there is no evidence that normal aging people require special supplements of vitamins, proteins, calcium, and other specific nutrients, diets may get out of balance when only a few restricted foods are eaten. Many elderly people are prone to restrict their diet to a few foods that are easily prepared and relatively cheap. Such a program can easily generate a variety of nutritional deficiencies. Special health foods represent primarily an added expense. All foods are basically healthy and the best protection against nutritional deficiencies is to consume a wide variety of foods under the same rules of nutrition that have been developed for the middle aged.

Another environmental factor which influences health and is under the direct control of the individual is cigarette smoking. There is no question that cigarette smoking is associated with an increase in the incidence of lung cancer and cardiovascular disease. It is, of course, true that some individuals who are heavy cigarette smokers never develop these diseases. Neither can it be shown that non-smokers never develop them. It is still a question of probability and the individual must decide for himself the extent to which he wishes to gamble with his own life-span.

Armed with knowledge gained from research about the general changes which occur with aging, individuals can take many active steps to minimize or even to avoid their effects. For example, sensory impairments that occur with advancing age can in many instances be corrected. The impairment in accommodation in vision can readily be corrected by proper fitting of bifocal lenses. Other visual impairments that make reading difficult can be compensated for simply by increasing the level of illumination. A 100-watt bulb to replace the 60-watt bulb can often make a world of difference. The decrease in night vision and increased susceptibility to glare may require the elimination of automobile driving at night but is not an unsurmountable obstacle. Hearing loss which is usually associated with aging can usually be compensated for by hearing aids. Dentures will replace missing teeth, and so on.

Lapses in immediate memory are both frustrating and irritating. It cannot be denied that they occur with increasing frequency as we get older. However, on a quantitative basis, the degree of memory loss with normal aging is not impressive. Although it has recently been reported that extracts of DNA and of chemicals which can be taken in the form of a pill result in substantial improvement of memory in elderly people, these reports must still be substantiated by extensive experimental work. I have no doubt that ultimately such aids will be developed. However, in the meantime we must rely on the usual devices such as writing things down or over-learning them by repetition. The fact has been shown that when older people are permitted to learn new material at their own pace, there is little difference between the learning ability of elderly Ss and young adults. Other aids to learning include actual speaking of the material or seeing and hearing it simultaneously.

In view of the known reduction in reserve capacity, it is important that aging people should reduce their exposure to unusual stresses. They should, however, maintain a program of planned activities that are both satisfying and meaningful. Oftentimes what passes as aging is nothing more than an atrophy of disuse. This is especially true within the sphere of mental activities. A good dictum would be to learn something new every day even if it comes under the heading of useless information. We might well adapt the Boy Scout dictum of " a good deed every day" to "a new deed every day" for the maintenance of health and vigor in the later years.

In summary I want to emphasize the expanding opportunities for the elderly. The combination of progress in basic research, medical skills, industrial technology, and social organization will increase the post-retirement period. This can represent the period of maximum fulfillment for the individual who seizes the opportunities and makes the most of them.

3 Research on aging: a frontier of science and social gain*

JAMES E. BIRREN, Ph.D.**

Research on aging has great implications for the health and well-being of adult man and the quality of his life in contemporary society. Few topics in the life sciences have more scope and significance than questions about the nature of aging in man and in other living systems. Having a national commitment to cultivate as high a proportion as possible of adults of sound body and mind who are able to function independently requires that we take definite steps to encourage research into the nature of aging. To carry out our commitment to the health and well-being of the population also requires that we strengthen the administrative context within which research is done so that we may gain from proved ideas at the earliest date. Research on aging finds itself in a new context. The public is restless for a higher quality of life for the adult and for the older person.

Several key questions in research on aging and a number of important national developments in programs for the aged demand attention. These questions can be distinguished as those of scientific problems, administrative organization of research, and public policy. New patterns of scientific effort and administration are needed—and are very slowly emerging, but all too slowly. Groups of scientists are becoming eager to study man's development over the

Reproduced from The Gerontologist 8:7-13, Spring, 1968.
*Adapted from a statement presented to the Senate Subcommittee on Government Research, Senator Fred Harris, chairman, October 24, 1966.
**Director, Rossmoor-Cortese Institute for the Study of Retirement and Aging, University of Southern California, Los Angeles, California.

life-span, including research on the interrelationships between physiological, psychological, and social factors in aging. If an optimum environment is to be created so individuals can realize their full biological and psychological potentials not only in youth and middle age but old age as well, we must have facts. We require an adequate national source of fundamental knowledge on which future services and sound administration of programs can be based. Right now planning for the aging is done on a fire brigade basis. We deal with specific problems, treat specific diseases, and build special facilities without fundamental understanding of the meaning of aging biologically, psychologically, and socially. This is a prescription for wasted effort.

How do we acquire these understandings? We need now to develop the concepts, the thinkers, the research facilities, the places of new therapy and observation. The nation has few germinating resources to undertake this assignment. I propose several policies and administrative arrangements to give needed strength to our national effort.

A. The federal government should establish university-based Institutes for Research on Aging at strategic places. We need headquarters not only for new research on aging but also to seize opportunities to add a gerontological perspective to biomedical research already in progress. The influences of the physical and social environment on aging should be included in the scope of research.

B. Research manpower is needed. Institutes for Research on Aging should serve as the centers for training the variety of investigators committed to studying influences on the life-span and the role of disease as well as physiological, psychological, and social changes of aging. What a loss if the need for aging studies was recognized years from now and society had to mark time until investigators could be trained.

C. We need lifelong systems of health maintenance. Technical excellence exists in medical and basic science specialties, but we need a multisystem approach in terms valuable to physicans and social thinkers—in terms of whole organisms and their environments. Missing is basic knowledge of how the human system becomes vulnerable as it ages.

D. Such a broad task requires new means of organizing scientific research since our usual administrative mechanisms simply are not geared to integrative studies of life. Research in aging has been faltering despite its potentials, despite indications that it could be at a take-off point. Administrative action should be considered now to: strengthen a national center for the study of aging within the National Institutes of Health on a scale that befits what we foresee as the national need for information on processes of aging; and establish, in conjunction with Institutes for Research on Aging, regional data banks organized to facilitate life-span research. These data banks would also be a natural part of a health "Preventicare" approach, that is, longitudinal multiphasic screening of populations.

Aging as a natural phenomenon

Research on aging is a vast frontier of science that has prospects for eventual gains in man's well-being.

Aging is a pervasive property of living things. Both plants and animals show characteristic changes with advancing age, such that one may recognize an individual as being "old." Being old implies that an animal has a short remaining life expectancy. Cuttings taken from old plants will show lower survival or less successful grafting than will cuttings from young members of the same species. Not only is aging commonly observed in other forms of life, its occurrence in man presents profound issues of research, administration, and personal values. Many animals in the wild state rarely have the chance to live to a late life; that is, they do not often live after the age of reproduction has ceased. However, when such animals are moved to a favorable environment they may survive longer and show a pattern of aging. Thus, animals that do not have the opportunity of showing aging in their predatory natural environments do have an inborn potential for aging which they can display if the environment becomes favorable.

This leads to the seemingly paradoxical point that aging is a product of favorable environments. In human terms, it is only in technologically advanced countries of the world that there is the privilege of large aging populations. In such countries, as in the United States, the intelligent layman along with the scientist asks the question, "What causes aging?"

Our concepts of aging have become refined in recent years as a result of the research of investigators from many different fields. In particular, no one dominating process of aging has been identified analogous, perhaps, to a single infectious disease or a single genetic factor. In fact, when describing man as a whole system, concepts like biological age, psychological age, and social age are useful to distinguish the various domains of function. As yet we know little about the interactions between biological, psychological, and social aging; but what we do know suggests their importance. As individuals we age biologically, psychologically, and socially. Our biological age refers to our position along a continuum from birth to death. Our psychological age refers to our adaptive capacities, our capacity to learn, remember, and respond effectively to our environment. Our social age refers to our habit systems or social roles. To some extent these are interdependent processes, and yet one knows of examples of individuals who may be biologically old and yet psychologically and socially young or, conversely, somebody who is biologically young and old psychologically and socially.

In the same sense, a little-used antique automobile may be a fine museum piece and in excellent running condition according to its original design and construction, and yet be socially antiquated in terms of the current demands of society. The current knowledge and information explosion can indeed result in earlier antiquation of individuals in the sense that their store of information has become dated. Other illustrations might be used to indicate that research on ging is a vast frontier of science, a frontier containing prospects for eventual gains for man's well-being, biologically, psychologically, and socially.

Man is a complex system which when it moves forward in time undergoes transformations in subsystems. Aging of various cells and of various organs and of various aspects of behavior do not proceed at the same rate. It is well to be sensitive to this point; for it would avail mankind little good if by prolonging life through the control of selected chronic diseases a population of mentally incompetent antiquarians would result. The nature of aging for the organism as a whole must be considered as well as the details of changes in individual organ systems.

Some biological considerations

A number of distinguished scientists have definitions of aging that have features in common. It is worthwhile to quote two of these definitions. Professor Philip Handler, a biochemist at Duke University, defined aging this way:

> Aging is the deterioration of a mature organism, resulting from time-dependent, essentially irreversible changes intrinsic to all members of a species, such that, with the passage of time, they become increasingly unable to cope with the stresses of the environment, thereby increasing the probability of death.

One notes in the definition an emphasis on the changes in the vulnerability in the host.

Dr. J. Maynard Smith defined aging this way:

> Aging processes are defined as those which increase the suspectibility of individuals as they grow older to the factors which may cause death.

These definitions of aging recognize the increased probability of death as a function of age of the organism.

The widespread occurrence of aging in nature suggested to earlier biologists that it must have had some selective value for the species. The reproduction of animals in the ascendancy of their physical maturity results in the young and vigorous propagating the species. This may be interpreted as meaning that aging is good for the species and undesirable for the individual. While it is quite likely that natural selection has played a role in aging, we have no real evidence of its influence.

It seems reasonable to conclude from the evidence that there has evolved in complex living systems a pattern of change which we call biological aging. Biological aging refers to a set of processes such that the individual organism becomes increasingly likely to die the longer he lives, even if he lives in a constantly favorable environment. The increased probability of dying with increasing age, called the force of mortality, has been studied in a number of species. While improving the environment will improve an individual's chances of survival, the form of the mathematical relationship between the probability of dying and age is not altered for populations. This has suggested that there is an inborn set of transformations of a biological nature in the aging individual which can to some extent be accelerated or delayed by the environment but not qualitatively altered. The conviction held by some biologists that there is an inborn tendency for species to age has been misinterpreted as implying inevitability about the longevity of mankind. This is a common misinterpretation of the scientist's need to isolate the basic processes of biological aging from the wide range of environmental influences on their expression.

The research question of whether there is one factor in aging has shifted to the contemporary question in research on aging of whether there are a few major processes of aging in man and other complex organisms or whether there is but a synchronization of many essentially independent biological processes of aging. It is quite possible that, in the course of evolution, unfavorable characteristics have been eliminated from early life by natural selection. Whereas in late life, that is after reproduction ceases, negative traits accumulate because it is difficult or impossible to eliminate them through natural selection. By this means there may have been developed a *precession* of favorable biological traits toward early life and a *recession* of negative traits toward later life. If this is so, the older the individual, the more likely he is to express some latent characteristic unfavorable to his survival.

One very important implication of such a hypothesis is that control or removal of one unfavorable factor in late life offers only minimum gain for survival since there are likely many other deleterious or lethal conditions that will appear at about the same time. If this is in fact the case, control of types of cancer, atherosclerosis, senile dementia, or other diseases in the aged would not therefore be expected to result in substantial prolongation of life as we have achieved by controlling single diseases in the young.

One clearly sees here profound long range implications for our concepts of human life that will arise from the pursuit of basic facts. Should it be found that the fundamental biological processes of aging are essentially independent processes, then the importance of control of the environment throughout the life-span will loom of even greater significance than the prospects of biological intervention in any particular disease that arises in late life. That is, a number of factors such as overnutrition, the amount of exercise and activity, and other influences that arise in our urban environments might affect the average rates of development of the independent aging processes. Depending on the results of future research, we will find out whether biological intervention into the isolated diseases of the aged will be as effective in improving man's longevity and health as improving the over-all quality of the environment in which he grows up and grows old.

At the present time, evidence of immortality of cells, derived from studies of tissue cultures, is under re-examination. Many, but not all, of the cells of the body turn over or are replaced, and one of the problems of the living organism is to provide a stability of function in the face of continuing turnover of cells. This point assumes significance with respect to aging since cells may possess a longer life-span than the organism system in which they are found. Put in terms of a scientific question, the issue is, do somatic cells age because of their intrinsic properties or do they age because of the changing body medium in which they are placed?

Modern research techniques in biology offer some exciting prospects for separating the importance of factors in aging. Organs may be transplanted from old and young donors to old and young hosts to determine, for example, whether the ovary itself ages or whether the ovary ages because of the condition of the organism. Similarly, it is now possible to transplant tissues and cells from old and young donors to old and young hosts. It is even possible to exchange the nuclei of old and young cells to tell us in the foreseeable future whether the genetic material of cells ages intrinsically or whether the cellular environment itself changes with age.

Other prospects for uncovering the importance of influences on rates of biological aging include the use of high and low environmental temperature to alter metabolic activity. The research laboratory can also be expected to tell us if there are age changes in the activity of specific cellular processes through the use of tracer substances.

In order to know where to place our emphasis in aging research, it is necessary to find out what proportion of the total phenomena of human aging is due to intrinsic aging properties of cells, to what extent it is the medium of the body in which cells are placed, and to what extent the complex phenomenon of aging is due to a breakdown of the integrating systems of the body, particularly the nervous system.

Cells of the nervous system assume particular significance in aging since, unlike many body cells, they are as old as the individual. Do nerve cells die eventually because they are old and show intrinsic changes, or do they die because they are part of an old individual? Whatever the mechanism involved, the failure to integrate functions of the body would ultimately produce a less efficient organism and one vulnerable to the strains of the environment.

There has been a habitual stance regarding aging that the smallest molecule in which one can demonstrate aging is necessarily the most basic point of attack for understanding the processes of aging. There is at present no clear basis for assuming that the major phenomenon of aging exists at any prescribed level of complexity of biological organization. For this reason, research must be encouraged at the molecular level, the cellular level, the organismic level, and the level of behavioral and social characteristics. One does not explain all the phenomena of psychological aging by biological processes, or similarly, an individual's social behavior is related to, but not completely determined by, his biological age and his change in psychological capacities. What causes aging, therefore, will be answered differently whether one has in mind how long people live, what their changes in mental ability and memory are, or what changes appear in their social behavior with advancing age. Almost without exception, contemporary students of aging would maintain that the processes of aging are multiple.

Considerations of the nervous system and psychological aging

In the course of evolution, a nervous system has developed which is in part organized on the basis of genetic characteristics of the species, and in part is organized on the basis of unique experience of the individual. Because this is true, biologists and behavioral scientists interested in the phenomenon of aging of whole organisms sooner or later must attend to the functional patterns acquired by the individual as the result of experience. Aging determines behavior; but behavior and the way behavior patterns are organized also determine the way the organism as a whole ages.

Here is an area of research in which aging and long-term consequences are explored with relation to the life-long occupations of individuals and their activities, interests, and particular patterns of emotional responses that they have developed over time. Cross cultural studies are also important since some of the characteristics we assume to be inherent to aging may indeed be the result of acquired behavior patterns or characteristics of our particular cultural environment.

Psychological aging concerns the limitations in adaptive capacities as individuals grow older. In this growing area of research recent evidence on large numbers of individuals suggests that there are behavioral characteristics which are predictive of the development of cardiovascular disease. There is thus the possibility of a feedback pattern in which a persistent behavior pattern predisposes to disease which results in damage to the nervous system which reduces the psychological capacities of the individuals. The behavioral precursors to high productivity in middle and late life need to be studied along with the behavioral dispositions to chronic disease. Some of the scientific questions have been defined, and the technology exists but we need research to secure the answers.

Social aging of man refers to his habit systems and social roles that he has acquired over his lifetime. Research on housing patterns for the aged indicates that modification of behavior even in the very aged occurs when the ease of social interactions is changed. This leads to questions about the principles that are needed for the scientific design of man's environment. The need for productive use of the competence that exists in our population of older adults depends upon our knowledge of the way patterns of social aging, including retirement, are established. There is much needed research in this area, particularly on the middle aged on whom much responsibility lies but about whom we know little.

Aging, longevity, and automated data systems

Closely related to research into the mechanisms of aging is research on the factors which can be used in predicting the longevity of an individual. If one compares the average length of life in different countries of the world, one will note significant differences. Also, within an individual country there is a wide range of individual differences in the length of life.

Hardin Jones compared the magnitude of a variety of environmental and health factors influencing the length of life. At the time he compared his data, about ten years ago, living in the country compared with living in the city would give an average additional length of life of five years. Having four grandparents who lived to 80 years would give a benefit of four years over the average life-span. The fact that having long-lived parents and grandparents confers a greater than average expected life-span is well known. What is not commonly recognized is such a hereditary contribution to longevity is at the present time less important quantitatively compared with environmental factors and other habits of living potentially under our control. Very likely, as the environment becomes favorably homogenous for all persons, hereditary aspects of longevity will become increasingly important. That is, a greater proportion of individual differences in life-span will be associated with differences in heredity and less to differences in the environment. For example, sex differences in longevity are expected to increase rather than decrease in future years.

The social scientist, however, sees a cultural correlation among elements of the environment. Just as genetic factors program development, so cultural factors determine the likelihood of incurring a given type of impairment as well as the consequences arising from it. Within the laboratory one may arbitrarily hold the environment constant while examining genetic or other biological influences on longevity. For man, however, both individual differences in heredity and in the environment are interacting. We need to break through the crust of customary thought so that we might examine with greater effectiveness biological as well as the social and environmental factors that do correlate with man's longevity.

Several areas of scientific activity need stimulation if we are to explore in adequate detail and to be able to predict the factors that determine man's longevity and well-being. These activities are: 1) the development of relevant mathematical models of interaction of health variables in a behavioral and social matrix; 2) the development of transducer systems involving bio-medical engineering and social and behavioral engineering for computer coupled data collection; 3) metasystem conceptualization of health, behavioral, and social variables. This leads to the development of models of critical systems and in a sense a "systems design of biological systems"; 4) investigations into the feasibility of time sampling and telemetry in community life for the collection of significant data related to health and behavioral change over the life-span; 5) development of systems of handling of longitudinal data on individuals so that the long-term outcomes of early antecedents can be explored.

An adequate research approach to phenomena of human aging requires a reorientation toward the collection and inter-relation of data. A block to progress has in part been a lack of conceptualization in which to fit data gathered by different specialists over the life-spans of individuals. If one is concerned with the well-being of individuals as they grow older from a physical, psychological, and social point of view, data will have to be collected by specialists in disciplines that normally do not work together. Some of the long-term antecedents to illness in middle age and late life either are due to or are encouraged by early life behavior and subsequently to occupational characteristics. Medicine, in dealing with the curative problems of disease, rarely has the time to deal with remote antecedents. Its stance is to deal with the most immediate biological precursor of the condition which sent the individual to the physician or hospital.

Medical science must take a longer-range view of the conceptual as well as the empirical requirements of longitudinal health systems. Such an approach includes the development of relevant mathematical models of interactions of health variables in a behavioral and social matrix. This has been described as a need for a metasystem conceptualization of health, behavioral, and social variables such that changes in health can be examined by auto-correlation of data remote in time from a present situation. Technological capability exists in medical specialties and in the many life sciences that can materially advance research in aging. A metasystem approach to human aging seems possible and needed for initiation in this decade.

Recent hearings in the United States Senate systematically explored the potentialities of multiphasic screening techniques in the detection of chronic illness. Witnesses before the Senate Sub-Committee on Health of the Elderly were almost universal in their conviction that automated annual health examinations would detect symptomatic or incipient illness at a stage that could result in great savings of suffering and financial costs. Complementary to such a "preventicare program" is the use of automated data collection and storage methods as part of longitudinal research studies on human functioning throughout the life-span. The possibilities that vital health data on large populations can be stored on magnetic tape and made available quickly are exciting. One may foresee the time when an individual's health record is filed nationally under his Social Security number and any medical facility which he approved could be granted access to magnetically stored life-span information by dialing the Social Security number.

Such a prospect might raise questions of invasion of privacy. However, such a system could exist by voluntary participation. I, for one, would feel much more secure if my personal physician could have access to the early life data from many medical histories that exist in the laboratories and clinics throughout the country in which physical examinations have been made on me. I would also recommend the inclusion of selected psychological and social data in such a history since I think it could be used for my family's and my benefit.

When issues of health and well-being are involved, there is little reason to regard blood characteristics as impersonal and personality predispositions to illness as personal. Both are personal sets of data that can be used for constructive research and individual care.

An overview

Because of the growth of scientific information and the vastness of potentially relevant data on aging, the scientist must be aided by a comprehensive information system which gives him immediate access to research information. In particular, the investigator in aging, since his subject matter cuts across disciplines, needs the assistance of a comprehensive information system. A center of aging information is necessary lest the scientist retreat and defend his integrity by unnecessarily scaling down the scope of problems he considers. The scientist will be forced to ignore information unless we make his task easier in the way of retrieving stored information for his use. The increase in the information load on the scientist in the field of aging can be appreciated by the fact that in the current decade more scientific literature will be published on the field of aging than in the entire previous history of the field. This is only a relative growth, however, since the field is just at take-off point. It does suggest, however, that this is a critical period in which to institute a coordinated information system. Whereas the major sin of past generations was not to seek knowledge, the sin of our current generation is to ignore information.

No matter how the scientist comes to view aging, contemporary society is faced with the responsibility for cultivating the health and well-being of a growing population of older adults. There are almost as many persons in the United States over the age 65 as there are total persons in the population of Canada, about nineteen million. The quality of life for older persons in the United States is being improved by administrative innovations, including the enaction of Medicare, improvements in the Social Security system, and the provision for special housing facilities for the aged. As we attempt to improve the quality of life for the adults of this country one may question whether we have an adequate national source of fundamental information on which to base future advances in the health and well-being of adult man and the quality of his life in contemporary society. Having a national commitment to cultivate the health and well-being of the population, we are desirous to take all steps to insure as high a proportion as possible of adults of sound body and mind and able to function independently. Among other efforts in our society this commitment requires that we encourage research into the nature of aging and also requires that we strengthen the administrative context within which research is done so that we may gain from proved ideas at the earliest date.

A changing national scene with higher expectations of the quality of life and the emergence of new social conditions of urban living has resulted in a changed definition of health. Not very long ago, good health was freedom from infectious disease. Now, particularly in relation to the aged, definitions of health are being broadened to include knowledge gained by the behavioral and social sciences as well as the bio-medical sciences. Our sophisticated technological society, in seeking a rational approach to the complex needs of an aging population is bringing into interaction the bio-medical sciences and the behavioral and social sciences. Both research and service to the aging require that we increasingly interrelate information from a broad array of sciences. This suggests that some attention needs to be given to ways of articulation of research, training, and services in the field of aging within our universities.

New types of scientist and administrator are emerging who have convictions that man does not function solely according to the arbitrary divisions of our sciences such as physiology, anatomy, and sociology. Groups of scientists are becoming eager to study man's development over the life-span, including such questions as how bio-medical factors influence the psychological well-being of the individual and how the social environment of the aging individual influences his health and psychological capacities. If an optimum environment is to be created in which individuals may develop and age in such a way as to realize their fullest potential, objective data must be gathered on many individuals over long portions of their life-span. Several Institutes for Research on Aging should be established for such purposes.

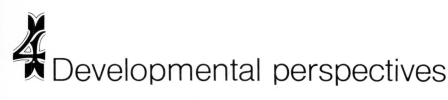

4 Developmental perspectives

BERNICE L. NEUGARTEN, Ph.D.*

As a developmental psychologist interested in creating a broadly-based developmental behavioral science, I should like to introduce my comments by saying that we need a psychology of the life-cycle—a psychology that will view the life-cycle as an appropriate unit for study, one that will encompass child development, adolescent development, adult development, aging, and the relationships between them. A psychology of the life-cycle would help to produce, in turn, a psychiatry of the life-cycle, one in which the relations between mental illness and mental health, pathology and non-pathology, would be examined always in light of development principles and age-related personality processes. Both the psychology and the psychiatry of the life-cycle are concerned with questions of continuities and discontinuities in the life history, or, in other words, with problems of stability and change in personality. Closely related is the problem of delineating the social and psychologic issues that arise at consecutive age periods in the life-cycle and differentiating those that are age-specific from those that are not. A second set of problems is concerned with individual differences between persons as they go from infancy to old age.

In considering developmental perspectives of the aging process, I want briefly to comment upon and to illustrate these problems. In each instance, I shall be drawing upon various sets of empirical studies carried on by myself and my colleagues in the Committee on Human Development at the University of Chicago, studies of large samples of middle-aged and older men and women, all of them living in the metropolitan areas of Kansas City or Chicago, and all of them living what we like to call "normal" lives.

Reproduced from Psychiatric Research Reports of the American Psychiatric Association 23:42-48, February, 1968.
*Professor of Human Development, University of Chicago, Chicago, Illinois.

Change in personality in middle and old age

While in many ways personality seems to remain relatively stable in middle and old age, in other ways measurable changes do occur. Because this field has as yet attracted only a few investigators, the picture is at best incomplete. Let me illustrate, however, from a series of studies based on various interview data and projective test data gathered from representative groups aged forty to eighty.

Significant and consistent age differences were found in both working-class and middle-class people in the perceptions of the self *vis-à-vis* the external environment and in their coping with impulse life. Forty-year-olds, for example, seem to see the environment as one that rewards boldness and risk-taking and to see themselves as possessing energy congruent with the opportunities perceived in the outer world. Sixty-year-olds, on the other hand, seem to perceive the world as complex and dangerous, no longer to be reformed in line with one's wishes, and the individual as conforming and less accommodating to outer-world demands.

Important differences exist between men and women as they age. Men seem to become more receptive to affiliative and nurturant promptings, women more responsive to and less guilty about aggressive and egocentric impulses. Men appear to cope with the environment in increasingly abstract and cognitive terms, women in increasingly affective and expressive terms. In both sexes older people move toward more egocentric, self-preoccupied positions and attend increasingly to control and satisfaction of personal needs.

With increasing old age, ego fuctions are turned inward, as it were. There is a change from active to passive modes of mastering the environment, and there is also a movement of energy away from an outer-world to an inner-world orientation, a change we called an increased "interiority" of personality.*

Whether or not this increased interiority has inherent as well as reactive qualities cannot yet be established—that is, whether these are time-related changes in personality that are reflections of biologic changes in the organism and are relatively independent of the environment, or whether the changes we see are in reaction to or in response to (or in anticipation of) changes in the social environment. It may be that in advanced old age biologically based factors become the pace-makers of personality changes; but this question awaits further disentangling of the effects of illness from the effects of aging *per se,* effects that presently are confounded in most older persons who are the subjects of psychologic research.

Some of our colleagues at Chicago broadened the interpretation of these findings, looked at some of our other findings regarding social participation patterns, and then set forth the "disengagement theory" (Cumming and Henry, 1961). That theory says, in essence, that people as they age withdraw from social and psychologic involvements in the environment at the same time that

---

*These findings have been described at greater length in Neugarten and associates (1964).

society withdraws its support from the aged person. In other words, there is a mutual process by which the individual shows a withdrawal phenomenon at the same time that, for various reasons, such as death of friends, death of spouse, or retirement, he suffers a series of social losses outside his control.

For the first part of the life span it appears that persons develop abilities, skills, and sets of psychologic mechanisms for dealing with the world, and their attention is given generally to managing the self and to practicing the techniques for dealing with an ever-widening world of experience. In middle age there is a reorganization and a re-evaluation of the self, a change in the quality of social interaction, and the beginning of a kind of interiority that involves a preoccupation with the inner life and new methods of dealing with impulse life. The major change-over probably begins in middle age, not in old age, although the processes are more characteristic of the old person. Thus, not all the withdrawal seen in very aged persons can be attributed to events that are happening in the family or in the work situation or in the kinds of losses that people experience as they age. Some of the withdrawal is probably "natural" in the sense that it is characteristic of most people as they move through the years from fifty to eighty.

The disengagement theory was, in part, a restatement of the everyday observation that persons as they grow old lose a great many of their social and psychologic ties to the environment. It was new in stating that aging is probably accompanied by some kinds of inner processes that make the loosening of social ties a relatively natural process.

The disengagement theory has been modified in the past few years, not only by its original authors, but by others of us who have continued to analyze the data on which it was based.* The modification has to do, not with those parts of the theory dealing with the loosening of social ties or psychologic withdrawal, but with those dealing with the postulated relationship between disengagement and well-being. It is now apparent on the whole, and contrary to the first statement of the disengagement theory, that persons who remain relatively active in the various social roles of family member, citizen, club member, friend, and so on, are the persons who report themselves most content with their lives. Thus, while it is likely that certain types of social loss and certain types of psychologic withdrawal are characteristic of most people as they grow old, it is simultaneously true that persons in whom these processes are most marked are not necessarily the happiest—as might have been predicted from a knowledge of the social values that characterize the American society.

In any case, the personality changes that I have mentioned are useful in the present context to illustrate that personality changes occur in the last half as well as in the first half of the life cycle and to illustrate the problems of charting

---

*The disengagement theory was first set forth by Cumming and Henry (1961). It has since been modified in such papers as Cumming (1963), Henry (1963), Havighurst, Neugarten, and Tobin (1964), and Neugarten (1965).

continuities and discontinuities from the point of view of a developmental perspective of the aging process.

Individual differences

The developmental psychologist is interested in discovering the similarities among people as they grow up and grow old; but he is interested also in discovering the differences. I have just illustrated a few of the personality changes that are characteristic of persons as they move from middle into old age; the same series of studies are useful to illustrate the great differences that exist.

There are many stereotypes in our society about old people growing more and more alike, but in our community samples we have been impressed with the way people grow more unlike. Indeed, it is probably an accurate view that differentiation continues throughout the lifetime and grows greater rather than less, until perhaps very advanced old age—perhaps at the very end of life—when biologic impairments may become so large that they limit and therefore narrow the variety of patterns of adaptation.

As researchers we tried to develop measures that would distinguish various phenomena: social role activity, personality pattern, and happiness (or life satisfaction).

One can, for instance, interview people at length and find out how much of their time is given to one after another social role—that is, how much time does the person spend in his role as spouse, or homemaker, or parent, or worker, or church member, or citizen, or club member, and so on—and one can say that one person is much higher in role performance than another person. At the same time, the researcher can develop a set of psychologic measures of how people structure their environments, what their inner feelings are, their self-concepts, and so on, and from these measures work out a system of personality types. Third, the researcher can measure how content or satisfied people are with their lives. If these are regarded as three somewhat independent measures, then one can study the relationships between these measures and, by so doing, describe the patterns of aging to be found in a community sample. In somewhat different words, we asked, what are the varieties of socio-psychologic patterns to be found? What situations produce greater satisfaction with life, given a certain kind of personality to start with?

Every individual is different from every other, of course, but we grouped individuals on the basis of similarities and differences on the three measures just mentioned. Let me describe the patterns of aging that emerged in persons who were aged seventy to seventy-nine. (The nature and variety of the patterns are somewhat different for younger and for older persons.)

The majority of our seventy-year-olds remained what we called *integrated* personalities: well-functioning persons with complex inner lives and intact cognitive abilities and competent egos. These persons were accepting of impulse life, over which they maintained a comfortable degree of control; they were flexible, open to new stimuli, mellow, mature. All these individuals, it happens, were rated high in life satisfaction. At the same time, they differed with regard to role activity: One group fell into a pattern we call the "reorganizers," who are the competent people engaged in a wide variety of activities. They are the optimum agers in some respects—at least in the American culture, where there is a high value placed on "staying young, staying active, and refusing to grow old." These are persons who substitute new activities for lost ones; who, when they retire from work, give time to community affairs or to church or to other associations. They reorganize their patterns of activity. A second pattern among the integrated personalities we call the "focused." These are integrated personalities, with high life satisfaction, who show only medium levels of activity. They have become selective in their activities, and they devote energy to one or two role areas. One such person, for instance, was a retired man who was now preoccupied with the roles of homemaker, parent, and husband. He had withdrawn from work and from club memberships and welcomed the opportunity to live a happy life with his family, seeing his children and grandchildren, gardening, and helping his wife with homemaking, which he had never done before. The third pattern we call the "disengaged." These are also integrated personalities, with high life satisfaction but low activity; persons who have voluntarily moved away from role commitments, not in response to external losses or physical deficits, but out of preference. These are self-directed persons, not shallow, with an interest in the world, but an interest that is not imbedded in a network of social interactions. They have high feelings of self-regard, just as do the first two groups mentioned, but they have chosen what might be called a "rocking chair" approach to old age—a calm, withdrawn, but contented pattern.

A second category includes the men and women whose personality type we call *armored* or *defended*. These are the striving, ambitious, achievement-oriented personalities, with high defenses against anxiety and the need to maintain tight controls over impulse life. This personality group provides two patterns of aging: one we call the "holding-on" pattern. This is the group to whom aging constitutes a threat, and who respond by holding on, as long as possible, to the patterns of their middle age. They are quite successful in their attempts, and thus maintain high life satisfaction with medium or high activity levels. These are persons who say, "I'll work until I drop," or "So long as you keep busy, you will get along all right." The other pattern we call the "constricted." These are persons busily defending themselves against aging, preoccupied with losses and deficits, dealing with these threats by constricting their social interactions and their energies and by closing themselves off from experience. They seem to structure their worlds to keep off what they regard as imminent collapse; and while this constriction results in low role activity, it works fairly well, given their personality pattern, to keep them high or medium in life satisfaction.

The third group of personalities is the *passive-dependent* type, among whom there are two patterns of aging. The "succorance-seeking" are those who have strong dependency needs and who seek responsiveness from others. These persons maintain medium levels of activity and medium levels of life satisfaction, and seem to maintain themselves fairly well so long as they have at least one or two other persons whom they can lean on and who meet their emotional needs. The "apathetic" pattern represents those persons in whom passivity is a striking feature of personality and who exhibit low role activity and medium or low life satisfaction. These are also "rocking chair" people, but with very different personality structures from those we have called the "disengaged." This apathetic pattern seems to occur in persons in whom aging probably has reinforced longstanding patterns of passivity and apathy. Here, for instance, was a man who, in the interviews, was content to let his wife do his talking for him, and a woman whose activities were limited entirely to maintaining her physical needs.

Finally, there is a group of *unintegrated* personalities who show a disorganized pattern of aging. These persons have gross defects in psychologic function, loss of control over emotions, and deterioration in thought processes. They maintain themselves in the community, but are low both in role activity and in life satisfaction.

These eight patterns do not exhaust all the varieties to be found in our group of seventy-year-olds, but given even this diversity, it is variation rather than similarity that is impressive. There is an implication, also, that the basic pattern of aging might be predicted for a given individual, given sufficient information about his personality and his general pattern of adaptation at an earlier age—say, at age fifty. (Given, also, of course, no overwhelming biologic accidents occurring to the subject.) It is, once again, the questions of continuity and discontinuity and of the range of individual differences that develop over time that preoccupy the developmental psychologist. To him, old age is not a separate and unique stage of life; to him the problems of the aged and the study of aging are to be seen within the complex of biologic, socio-cultural, and personal variation that provides the context for studying all stages of life.

REFERENCES

Cumming, E. 1963. Further thoughts on the theory of disengagement. Int. Soc. Sci. J., **15**:337-393.

Cumming, E. and Henry, W. E. 1961. Growing old. New York: Basic Books.

Havighurst, R. J., Neugarten, B. L., and Tobin, S. S. 1964. Disengagement, personality and life satisfaction in the later years. In P. F. Hansen (Ed.), Age with A Future. Copenhagen: Munksgaard, pp. 419-425.

Henry, W. E. 1963. The theory of intrinsic disengagement. Paper read at the International Research Seminar on Social and Psychological Aspects of Aging, Markaryd, Sweden, August, 1963.

Neugarten, B. L. 1965. Personality and patterns of aging. J. of Psychology of the University of Nijemegen (Gawein), **13**:249-256.

Neugarten, B. L., and associates. 1964. Personality in Middle and Late Life. New York: Atherton.

The functional assessment of elderly people

M. POWELL LAWTON, Ph.D.*

Psychological testing originated in the need of school teachers to look objectively at the ability of pupils with different life experiences. Teachers were keenly aware of the biases and extraneous influences that might enter into their judgment of the educability of a youngster. Thus, Alfred Binet began the search for a standardized measure of intelligence, and originated the concept of the intelligence quotient. Although the I.Q. is going through hard times right now, the fact remains that systematic evaluation of the behavior and inner processes of the older person is an indispensable aid to the proper treatment of the aged. Techniques for assessing the functioning of older people have not yet attained the scientific sophistication of the I.Q. measurement, but they are available in a nascent form that can be of great help to the medical practitioner. This article outlines some of the rationale for assessment, with the theoretical basis, and describes some of the available techniques.

Functional assessment, in this context, means any systematic attempt to measure objectively the level at which a person is functioning, in any of a variety of areas such as physical health, quality of self-maintenance, quality of role activity, intellectual status, social activity, attitude toward the world and toward self, and emotional status. Not all these areas, strictly speaking are in the domain of mental health. However, since the unity of body and mind is nowhere better exemplified than in the aging person, it seems essential to consider every area that may possibly affect the older person's emotional state. One of the clearest and most recurrent findings in all gerontological research is the mutual

Reproduced from Journal of the American Geriatrics Society 19:465-481, June, 1971.
*Research Psychologist, Philadelphia, Geriatric Center, 5301 Old York Road, Philadelphia, Pennsylvania 19141.

interdependence of physical state, adaptive behavior, and emotional state. For example, in study after study, the best predictor of the morale of older people is their physical health. Thus each of the major subsystems of human function may properly be regarded as relevant to emotional health. END.

The busy practitioner may well wonder why he should take valuable time to use evaluational techniques. The case for formalized assessment is multifaceted:

1. Assessment insures that all areas of functioning are considered in treating the patient. In this sense, a series of devices to measure functioning in a number of different areas serves much as does a shopping list. It guards against forgetting to look at potentially important assets or liabilities. This procedure also reminds us of the strengths of the individual, as well as his weaknesses.

2. Assessment of all areas gives a more complete picture of the living, functioning person. The pattern of assets and deficits may be more significant than any specific disability. Poor mental performance in a person who is marginally competent in most other areas probably means gross general impairment. In a person whose functioning checks out well in social and instrumental areas, low mental performance may mean poor hearing, language difficulty, test anxiety, or some other nonintellectual disability.

3. Formalized assessment techniques provide some objective evidence for the clinical impression. The standardization of such measures involves much effort to achieve clarity of language, definition of terms, and instructions for questioning or rating. This somewhat compulsive exercise reduces the observer's errors and discourages bias.

4. Communication to others is facilitated. Once the spadework is done, it becomes increasingly easy to tell another member of the treatment team, or another doctor, about the patient's condition. Almost everyone has some comprehension of the meaning of a given I.Q. The physician can communicate a great deal by simply stating a cardiac patient's rating on the American Heart Association's classification system. Judicious sharing of the content of some of the assessment devices with the family may convey the magnitude of the patient's ability or disability better than can the physician's extended verbal comments.

5. The results of treatment are more easily assessed. In some cases, the patient can tell you that his symptom has disappeared, or the physician knows that the disappearance of a certain sign is clear evidence of improvement. Many disabilities have indicators that are less clear-cut, however. Physical medicine has long recognized that in order to reflect change over time in the effectiveness of functioning, small-scale measures of specific behaviors are required. Such information fed back to the physician and other members of a therapeutic team in easily communicable form is a valuable guide for what to do next. Such longitudinal measures may also positively motivate those who give treatment. If they have objective evidence that their therapy is successful, they are more likely to sustain their effort.

6. Formalized assessment helps the practitioner monitor his own professional techniques. By looking at specific functions of his patient, he is forced to think about specific therapeutic measures that he can apply. Thus he is made aware of lacks in his own information or technical skill, and will be motivated to fill the void.

I have found it convenient to conceive of behavior in a hierarchy, ranging from relatively low complexity (the level of organ function, or disease) to the highest complexity (social behavior).[1] Inner states, in contrast, are related, but not on the same continuum.[2] In this article I discuss assessment techniques suited to each of these levels, emphasizing wherever possible those that are relatively available and easy to use by the practitioner treating older people. For most of these techniques, data are not yet at hand for establishing cut-off points to indicate what sort of action one might take. Generally, each user must establish a frame of reference in his own mind as to how low or how high a given score is for his own purposes, and for the type of patient he works with.

Physical health

There is no satisfactory global index of physical health. Health is a concept far too complex to be represented by a single number. Lawton, Ward and Yaffe[3] analyzed statistically 52 separate measures of health, hoping to obtain a smaller number of indicators. Even with the use of factor analysis to reduce the number, eight to ten separate health factors remained. It was clear that the determination of health depends upon whether one questions the subject or the doctor, or it depends upon available health records. Health behavior and health anxiety are also important aspects. The results of our factor analysis demonstrated clearly that no single index can properly represent an individual's health.

On the theory that diagnosis itself conveys some information about the subject's health, Wyler, Masuda and Holmes[4] had 117 physicians rate 126 conditions for "seriousness." They established a consensus rank order ranging from dandruff as the least serious to leukemia as the most serious. Theoretically, with this list in hand, one could sum the rankings of diagnoses pertaining to a given patient and obtain a rank sum indicating how ill he is. A still better approach, not yet established to my knowledge, would be to allow a severity rating for each condition and to sum the combined rank-times-severity ratings.

Burack,[5] in the first section of a wide-range assessment for a treatment scale, classifies chronic and acute conditions into four categories, the major dimensions being: a) relevancy to the "immediate clinical state," and b) the outlook for life expectancy. His definitions are broad enough to augment the accuracy of rating, though still concise and clear enough for ready use.

The difficulties of representing health in any unitary way have led most researchers to the easier task of measuring disability. One of the older methods of measuring disability is the Veterans Administration system of taking an individual's total functioning as a baseline, and estimating the percentage reduction in total function attributable to each diagnosed condition. Such disabilities may range from zero to 100 per cent, and are summative. Thus, a person might be considered disabled by an anxiety state to the extent that his social functioning was reduced by 20 per cent; residual pain from a shrapnel wound might occasionally be mildly exacerbated, with 10 per cent reduction in efficiency; and a burn scar would be diagnosable but not disabling. His total disability would then be 30 per cent. This system has been used successfully by the major interdisciplinary gerontology project at Duke University.[6]

Sokolow et al.[7] also have worked with percentages of disability in rating several systems, including the social and psychiatric, and combining them in *a priori* mathematical form.

Many other global measures of functional health have been used. The most global have the primary advantage of being easy to use. Conceptually they are, at best, a mixture. One such scale developed by Waldman and Fryman[8] for use at the Philadelphia Geriatric Center (PGC) is reproduced in Table 1. It is a six-point scale. The highest number under which any lettered statement is checked determines the rating. As a general guide to placement, this is a very useful scale. Among the PGC staff who know the scale, a rating of "Two" communicates a fairly accurate picture of an individual's general capability: he may need institutional care, but not necessarily in a medical setting. A patient rated "One" probably does not need such care, but a "Six" can be treated only with full hospital care.

Physical self-care

The disadvantage of global ratings is that they permit more observer bias, less directed thinking about the nature of the disability, and particularly the confusing necessity of weighing a disability in one area (a diagnosable disease, for instance) against an ability in a different area (e.g., the ability to walk normally). This is the old "peaches and pears" problem. Therefore, it is most rewarding to break down disability into its component parts, of which the ability to take care of oneself physically is the most basic. The so-called "activities of daily living schedule" (ADL) is used in most rehabilitation settings to rate objectively how independently and adequately the patient dresses, grooms himself and takes care of toileting. The tradition that each institution makes its own ADL schedule, has resulted in instruments of similar content that vary widely in psychometric sophistication.

Katz et al.[9] developed a scale that meets adequate psychometric criteria to measure whether a patient is fully dependent in bathing, dressing, going to the toilet, changing body location, feeding, and continence. They collected a great deal of validation data, and the scale is arranged in accordance with an underlying theory of physical rehabilitation. Lowenthal[10] reported a similar scale, with the advantage that independence is not an all-or-nothing measure; the scale allows for measuring degrees of dependence. Her Langley-Porter Physical

Table 1. Physical classification

I. a. Capable of unlimited and unsupervised activity.
   b. Fully ambulatory; able to go about the city independently in safety.
   c. Has no physical condition requiring medical supervision or closeness to emergency medical care.
   d. No evidence of heart disease in any form.
   e. No evidence of prior cancer except cured skin cancer.
   f. No complaints except those which cannot be related to any known disease entity.

II. a. Capable of moderate activity; ambulatory without supervision for activities in his own home or immediate vicinity.
    b. Can manage without help for care, and otherwise requires minimal supervision.
    c. Physical condition may require medical supervision, but frequent or special treatment or closeness to medical or nursing care not required.
    d. May have had a previous illness which has left no residuals, e.g., healed myocardial infarction without angina or ECG abnormalities other than healed infarctions, cancer with no evidence of recurrence, or mild diabetes (diet-controlled).

III. a. Limited capabilities.
     b. Dependent on others for bedmaking and baths and general supervision of activities.
     c. May or may not need a walking aid (cane) but can carry on routine activities without additional personal service.
     d. Generally requires escort on the outside.
     e. May require regular periodic medical care; availability of emergency medical or nursing care desirable.
     f. These people have moderate incapacities such as angina, arthritis which does not limit them to a wheel-chair, chronic respiratory disease, or diabetes requiring medication.

IV. a. Limited capabilities requiring assistance for personal care and daily living activities.
    b. Must be in a protected environment because of need for general nursing supervision.
    c. Closeness to emergency medical care desirable.
    d. Requires periodic medical care at close intervals.
    e. These persons are practically housebound.
    f. Angina or intermittent heart disease limits physical capacities, arthritis prevents ambulation, and there are severe hearing or visual impairments, but these patients still have the capacity to be independent for daily activities after orientation.

V. a. Chronically ill and confined to the vicinity of their own rooms.
   b. Require a large amount of personal service, and constant supervision.
   c. Should be near their own dining and toilet areas, and have a nurse on call at all times.
   d. Physical condition requires 24-hour nursing care or intensive medical treatment.

VI. Persons requiring hospital-type care:
    a. Bed patients requiring intensive medical and nursing care.
    b. Patients with infectious or contagious disease.

Table 2. Physical Self-Maintenance Scale

	Score
A. *Toilet*	
1. Cares for self at toilet completely; no incontinence	1
2. Needs to be reminded, or needs help in cleaning self, or has rare (weekly at most) accidents	0
3. Soiling or wetting while asleep, more than once a week	0
4. Soiling or wetting while awake, more than once a week	0
5. No control of bowels or bladder	0
B. *Feeding*	
1. Eats without assistance	1
2. Eats with minor assistance at meal times, with help in preparing food or with help in cleaning up after meals	0
3. Feeds self with moderate assistance and is untidy	0
4. Requires extensive assistance for all meals	0
5. Does not feed self at all and resists efforts of others to feed him	0
C. *Dressing*	
1. Dresses, undresses and selects clothes from own wardrobe	1
2. Dresses and undresses self, with minor assistance	0
3. Needs moderate assistance in dressing or selection of clothes	0
4. Needs major assistance in dressing but cooperates with efforts of others to help	0
5. Completely unable to dress self and resists efforts of others to help	0
D. *Grooming* (neatness, hair, nails, hands, face, clothing)	
1. Always neatly dressed and well-groomed, without assistance	1
2. Groom self adequately, with occasional minor assistance, e.g., in shaving	0
3. Needs moderate and regular assistance or supervision in grooming	0
4. Needs total grooming care, but can remain well groomed after help from others	0
5. Actively negates all efforts of others to maintain grooming	0
E. *Physical ambulation*	
1. Goes about grounds or city	1
2. Ambulates within residence or about one block distant	0
3. Ambulates with assistance of (check one): *a* ( ) another person, *b* ( ) railing, *c* ( ) cane, *d* ( ) walker, or *e* ( ) wheelchair: 1 __ gets in and out without help 2 __ needs help in getting in and out	0
4. Sits unsupported in chair or wheelchair, but cannot propel self without help	0
5. Bedridden more than half the time	0
F. *Bathing*	
1. Bathes self (tub, shower, sponge bath) without help	1
2. Bathes self, with help in getting in and out of tub	0
3. Washes face and hands only, but cannot bathe rest of body	0
4. Does not wash self but is cooperative with those who bathe him	0
5. Does not try to wash self, and resists efforts to keep him clean	0

Self-Maintenance Scale was modified by Lawton and Brody for easier institutional use.[11] Table 2 shows these scales. Each scale, A through F, is checked to indicate the patient's status regarding each function. His total score may range from zero to 6, one point being given for each function in which the subject obtains the most independent score. Thus, the score communicates the general level of his self-maintaining capacity. The specifics of his abilities and disabilities are conveyed by reference to the point on each scale where his competence lies. Norms usable for individual decision-making do not exist yet. However, rough guidelines may be found in data from 343 cases; in this series, applicants to a home for aged had a mean score of 4.1, patients admitted to a mental hospital reception center had a mean score of 3.5, and protective-custody patients had a mean score of 2.0. Thus, a zero score would probably preclude adjustment outside an institution which provides very close supervision, but a score in the range 2-6 would allow placement in a home for the aged (depending upon the amount of service available).

Instrumental activities of daily living

Paid work is the best example of an instrumental activity. After retirement, other daily tasks become most relevant to the living of a minimally adequate social life. Lawton and Brody[11] named a set of eight such tasks the Instrumental Activities of Daily Living (IADL) as shown in Table 3. One can live outside an institution without being able to perform some of them satisfactorily. However, the more these abilities are impaired, the more will formal or family-administered services be required to maintain the person in the community. The IADL is also scaled as is the self-maintenance scale, but in the IADL, a person receives a score of 1 for each item labelled A through H if his competence attains some minimal level *or higher.* Thus, for item A, telephone use, the subject receives one tally if he can answer the telephone, or do better; on item B, however, he gets a tally only if he can take care of all shopping needs independently. Items C and D (cooking and housekeeping) are relatively specific to the female role and are therefore not included in scoring for males. We have tested fewer subjects on this scale than are requisite for even minimal use for screening, and therefore recommend that each user treat the scale qualitatively at first, until he gets some idea of how his own patients are responding. The examiner fills out the scale on the basis of the maximal amount of knowledge he has about the patient from the patient himself, informants, and recent records.

Mental status

Mental status in its traditional usage refers to the capacity to be oriented for time, place and person, to remember, and to perform intellectual tasks of varying degrees of difficulty. Traditional psychological testing with standardized tests such as the Wechsler Adult Intelligence Scale are the most satisfactory measures of mental status, provided the person is attentive, educated at least to a

Table 3. Scale for Instrumental Activities of Daily Living

Males' score		Females' score
	A. *Ability to use telephone*	
1	1. Operates telephone on own initiative; looks up and dials numbers, etc.	1
1	2. Dials a few well-known numbers	1
1	3. Answers telephone but does not dial	1
0	4. Does not use telephone at all	0
	B. *Shopping*	
1	1. Takes care of all shopping needs independently	1
0	2. Shops independently for small purchases	0
0	3. Needs to be accompanied on any shopping trip	0
0	4. Completely unable to shop	0
	C. *Food preparation*	
	1. Plans, prepares and serves adequate meals independently	1
	2. Prepares adequate meals if supplied with ingredients	0
	3. Heats and serves prepared meals, or prepares meals but does not maintain adequate diet	0
	4. Needs to have meals prepared and served	0
	D. *Housekeeping*	
	1. Maintains house alone or with occasional assistance (e.g., heavy-work domestic help)	1
	2. Performs light daily tasks such as dish-washing and bed-making	1
	3. Performs light daily tasks but cannot maintain acceptable level of cleanliness	1
	4. Needs help with all home maintenance tasks	1
	5. Does not participate in any housekeeping tasks	0
	E. *Laundry*	
	1. Does personal laundry completely	1
	2. Launders small items; rinses socks, stockings, etc.	1
	3. All laundry must be done by others	0
	F. *Mode of transportation*	
1	1. Travels independently on public transportation or drives own car	1
1	2. Arranges own travel via taxi, but does not otherwise use public transportation	1
0	3. Travels on public transportation when assisted or accompanied by another	1
0	4. Travel limited to taxi or automobile, with assistance of another	0
0	5. Does not travel at all	0
	G. *Responsibility for own medication*	
1	1. Is responsible for taking medication in correct dosages at correct time	1
0	2. Takes responsibility if medication is prepared in advance in separate dosages	0
0	3. Is not capable of dispensing own medication	0

Table 3. Scale for Instrumental Activities of Daily Living—cont'd

Males' score		Females' score
	H. *Ability to handle finances*	
1	1. Manages financial matters independently (budgets, writes checks, pays rent and bills, goes to bank); collects and keeps track of income	1
1	2. Manages day-to-day purchases, but needs help with banking, major purchases, etc.	1
0	3. Incapable of handling money	0

Table 4. Mental Status Questionnaire

1. Where are we now? (Correct name of place)
2. Where is this place? (Correct city)
3. What is today's *date*? (Day of month)
4. What month is it?
5. What year is it?
6. How old are you?
7. What is your birthday? (Month)
8. What year were you born?
9. Who is President of the United States?
10. Who was President before him?

Scores: 0–2 CBS absent or mild.
3–8 CBS moderate.
9–10 CBS severe.

minimal level, conversant in English, unimpaired in senses, and accepts the testing situation as one worth his cooperation. These provisos eliminate many elderly subjects; moreover, the services of a psychologist are not always available. Also, the task is frequently one of discriminating between severe mental impairment and moderate impairment, which cannot be accomplished with many of the standardized tests. To meet this need, Kahn, Pollack and Goldfarb[12] designed the ten-item Mental Status Questionnaire (MSQ) shown in Table 4. With such a simple series of items, the examiner can compensate for the subject's deficiencies in language, sensory reception, attention, or motivation by mechanisms such as repetition, speaking loudly, translating, and working hard to mobilize the subject's attention for a brief span of time. The authors have tested enough people with this questionnaire to be able to identify the gradations of probable chronic brain syndrome noted in Table 4. Independent psychiatric examinations of 328 subjects indicated that only 12 per cent of older patients making no errors or only 1 or 2 errors were certifiable as suffering from mental illness by New York State standards, whereas 78 per cent of those making 9 or 10 errors were certifiable. This MSQ is in wide use as an aid to understanding just how much of a patient's exhibited difficulty is attributable to chronic brain syndrome. "Normal" senescence does not result in a lowering of scores on the MSQ, nor do most neurotic conditions. Nonorganic psychoses (depression, schizophrenia) may or may not result in lowered scores, but other indicators can usually determine whether it is a functional psychosis that is impairing performance.

There are many other approaches to the assessment of functional mental status. The MSQ will not discriminate above a minimal level of competence. However, the physician in practice is less likely to have to distinguish whether his older patient is superior or only average in intelligence. Such a question may be relevant in extended counseling, vocational redirection, or psychiatric rehabilitation. In these instances, a complete series of psychodiagnostic tests should be performed by a clinical psychologist.

Social roles and activities

The more complex the behavior, the more difficult it is to measure successfully. Social behavior on a very low level can be measured fairly accurately, as in the author's[13] adaptation of a Minimal Social Behavior Scale (MSBS).[14] This test situation presents the subject with a number of basic social stimuli (such as a greeting, an invitation to be seated, a chance to do a favor, and so on), and the responses are scored for their social appropriateness. Table 5 shows the 25-item geriatric version of the MSBS. Norms are not available for this test, but a rough idea of how scores run may be gained from the fact that the average score for relatively intact geriatric mental patients was 22, whereas the average score for impaired and uncooperative patients was 15.

For behavior within the normal range, the most-used instrument over the years has been the Chicago Activity and Attitude Inventory.[15] The first part of this inventory obtains information on the subject's behavior in the areas of health, friendship and family contacts, leisure-time use, economic security, and religion. The inventory is out of print, but may be reproduced from the book; information on the manual, with norms for large numbers of older people, may be obtained from its author.* With these norms, one can compare a given older person's level of activity with that of other people roughly comparable in status to the subject. The one major difficulty with the Inventory is that it is set up in "test" format, so that the subject fills out his own responses. Both the test format and the language in which the items are phrased are likely to cause some response problems in older people below a moderate level of sophistication and mental competence.

---

*Robert Havighurst, Ph.D., Judd Hall, University of Chicago, Chicago, Ill. 60637.

Table 5. Minimal Social Behavior Scale

A. E. goes to S. and introduces himself: *"I am* _____ *, Mrs.* _____ *. I'm glad to meet you,"* extending hand.
  1) Score + if any discernible response to greeting
  2) Score + if response is verbal and appropriate
  3) Score + if S. offers hand to E.

B. E. says either (a) *"Won't you have a seat?"* or (b) *"May I sit with you for a while?"* depending on whether S. is brought to E. or E. comes to S.
  4) Score + if (a) s. sits without urging, or (b) S. assents or acknowledges E.'s comment

C. E. says *"How are you today?"*
  5) Score + if any discernible response to question
  6) Score + if response is verbal and appropriate

D. E. drops pencil by pushing it off desk, ostensibly by accident. If S. does not pick up pencil spontaneously, E. says *"Would you pick up the pencil for me?"*
  7) Score + if S. picks up pencil at all
  8) Score + if S. picks up pencil spontaneously

E. E. says *"I have something I want to show you."* E. holds in front of S., Figure A of the Bender-Gestalt test (E. may draw for S. a circle being touched by one corner of a square).
  9) Score + if S. looks at Bender card

F. *"Here is a pencil."* E. offers it to S., puts paper in front of S., and says, *"I would like you to copy this drawing on this paper."*
  10) Score + if S. accepts pencil without further urging
  11) Score + if S. makes any mark on paper
  12) Score + if S. draws an appropriate circle and 4-sided figure

G. E. says *"How are you getting along?"*
  13) Score + if any discernible response to the question
  14) Score + if the response is verbal and appropriate

H. E. crumples a scrap of paper and tosses it at a wastebasket previously placed next to S., purposely missing.
  15) Score + if S. spontaneously picks up paper and deposits it in wastebasket

I. E. says *"I have a few questions I would like to ask you."* (E. administers questions 1-10 of Kahn-Goldfarb Mental Status Questionnaire.)
  16) Score + if S. makes any verbal response , irrespective of content, to all questions 1-10

J. E. places a magazine in front of S. and busies himself with writing on pad while saying, *"I'll be busy a minute."*
  17) Score + if S. turns at least one page of magazine

K. E. rises and extends hand, saying *"Thank you very much Mr(s).* _____ *."*
  18) Score + if S. acknowledges E.'s departure either verbally or with gesture

L. The remainder of the items are based on E.'s judgment of the behavior of the patient throughout the interview:
  19) Score + unless inappropriate grimaces or mannerisms are readily apparent
  20) Score + if the patient at any time looks E. in the eye
  21) Score + unless S. obviously appears to avoid E.'s gaze at all times, or stares at E. fixedly
  22) Score + unless S. sits in a bizarre position or is in constant motion or is nearly motionless
  23) Score + unless S.'s clothes are obviously disarranged, unbuttoned, or misbuttoned
  24) Score + unless S. is drooling or nasal mucus is visible or food deposits are conspicuous on clothes or face
  25) Score + unless S. attempts to move away from E. before termination of interview with explanation

Havighurst has also developed a set of Role Activity Ratings by which an informant or professional who knows the subject well can rate activity in a number of relatively specific roles such as grandparent, parent, extended family member, business club member, or civic participant. In one form, the level of competence with which the subject performs the role tasks is rated.[16] In the other and slightly more extended form, the energy expended in the role behavior, rather than its quality, is rated.[17] Norms for the latter are available for older people in several countries.

Attitudes, morale, and life satisfaction

On the level of inner psychological state, the usual standard assessment instruments such as the Minnesota Multiphasic Personality Inventory, the Edwards Personal Preference Schedule, or the Maudsley Personality Inventory are quite unsuitable for many geriatric patients. They are too long, and the language of even the simplest of them (the MMPI) taxes the comprehension of enough patients to preclude their routine use. Because of these difficulties, a number of scales have been designed specifically for older people. There is not enough space here to discuss adequately and to distinguish among the concepts of attitudes, morale, life satisfaction, adjustment, and positive mental health in older people. Excellent considerations of these issues have been presented by Rosow[18] and Havighurst,[19] and a review of some work in this area was made by Lawton.[20]

One approach to the measurement of attitude is that of Cavan et al.—the Chicago Activity and Attitude Inventory.[15] The section on activities described above is followed by a section in which the subject is asked questions regarding his attitudes and satisfaction with each major field activity.

The simplest measure of morale, and one that has been found useful in a large number of gerontological studies, is the Kutner Morale Scale, shown in Table 6.[21] The subject receives one tally for each item answered in the direction indicated in Table 6. Among the 500 subjects of Kutner et al., approximately one-third each received scale scores classifiable as high, medium, and low respectively. This scale can be read and answered by the subject, or an examiner can read him the questions. Its brevity makes the Kutner scale an admirable instrument for brief assessment. However, its content is limited, its language ponderous, and its brevity a liability in terms of its capacity to measure accurately a complex concept.

Neugarten, Havighurst and Tobin,[22] in connection with the Kansas City Study of Adult Life,[23] assembled a set of questions that seemed central for adjustment to living during old age. Using information obtained from depth psychological interviews as a validating criterion, they painstakingly devised two measures of adjustment: 1) Life Satisfaction Index A, and 2) Life Satisfaction Index B. The former scale has been analyzed further and its length reduced to 13 items, as shown in Table 7—the Life Satisfaction Index Z.[24] Among the normal

Table 6. Kutner Morale Scale

Question	Response alternatives	Score
1. How often do you feel that there's just no point in living—often, sometimes, or hardly ever?	Often	0
	Sometimes	0
	Hardly ever	1
2. Things just keep getting worse and worse for me as I get older	Agree	0
	Disagree	1
3. How much do you regret the chances you missed during your life to do a better job of living—not at all, somewhat, or a good deal?	Not at all	1
	Somewhat	0
	A good deal	0
4. All in all, how much unhappiness would you say you find in life today?—almost none; some, but not very much; a good deal?	Almost none	1
	Some, but not very much	0
	A good deal	0
5. On the whole, how satisfied would you say you are with your way of life today? Would you say—very satisfied, fairly satisfied, or not very satisfied?	Very satisfied	1
	Fairly satisfied	0
	Not very satisfied	0
6. How much do you plan ahead the things you will be doing next week or the week after? Would you say you make—many plans, a few plans, or almost none?	Many plans	1
	A few plans	1
	Almost none	0
7. As you get older, would you say things seem to be better or worse than you thought they would be?	Better	1
	Worse	0
	Same	0

Scores: 0–2 Low morale.
          3–4 Medium.
          5–6 High morale.

aged, Wood, Wylie, and Sheafor[24] found that scores of 0-12 indicated low morale, 13-21 moderate, and 22-26 high morale. Norms are not available for many groups, however, such as psychiatric patients, and the user must again establish his own frame of reference. The longer version may be reproduced from the original article,[22] and studies using a variety of types of aged people have been reported.

Lawton was dissatisfied with the language, the sometimes difficult response format, and the lack of comprehensiveness of content of other measures of morale, and assembled a group of items with these considerations in mind.[20] The items found to be valid predictors of rated adjustment were subjected to a factor analysis, resulting in the Philadelphia-Geriatric-Center Morale Scale shown in Table 8. A total score is obtained by summing all the "plus" responses. The

Table 7. Life Satisfaction Index Z

	Score		
	Agree	?	Disagree
1. As I grow older, things seem better than I thought they would be	2	1	0
2. I have gotten more breaks in life than most of the people I know	2	1	0
3. This is the dreariest time of my life	0	1	2
4. I am just as happy as when I was younger	2	1	0
5. These are the best years of my life	2	1	0
6. Most of the things I do are boring or monotonous	0	1	2
7. The things I do are as interesting to me as they ever were	2	1	0
8. As I look back on my life, I am fairly well satisfied	2	1	0
9. I have made plans for things I'll be doing a month or a year from now	2	1	0
10. When I think back over my life, I didn't get most of the important things I wanted	0	1	2
11. Compared to other people, I get down in the dumps too often	0	1	2

average score obtained by 500 tenants of specialized housing developments for the elderly was about 13. Scores ranging from 10 through 17 can be considered usual, whereas scores of 9 or below raise a distinct question as to whether the person is in some psychological distress, or badly mismatched with his total environmental situation. The PGC Morale Scale deliberately phrases questions in an oversimplified way, and forces responses into an "either-or" format so as to be easy for almost everyone to answer. It may be filled out by the subject himself, or read and marked by an examiner. The results of the statistical analysis (not presented here) indicated that the test was successful in measuring diverse aspects of morale, such as anxiety, loneliness, pessimistic outlook, dissatisfaction with the environment, and negative attitude toward aging.

Psychiatric status

There are, by now, hundreds of formal devices for rating psychiatric status from a pathology-oriented point of view. A number of these can be used with the aged, but few have been designed specifically with the common symptoms of this group in mind. This lack is almost complete in the case of formalized psychiatric ratings designed for the patient living in the community. Most of the schedules now in use are, unfortunately, designed with the institutionalized patient in mind. The best of these is very long and still in an experimental stage—the Mental Status Schedule, Geriatric Supplement, of Spitzer et al.[25] All

Table 8. Philadelphia-Geriatric-Center (PGC) Morale Scale

Question	Response alternatives	Score
1. Things keep getting worse as I get older	No	1
	Yes	0
2. I have as much pep as I did last year	Yes	1
	No	0
3. How much do you feel lonely?	Not much	1
	A lot	0
4. Little things bother me more this year	Yes	0
	No	1
5. I see enough of my friends and relatives	Yes	1
	No	0
6. As you get older you are less useful	Yes	0
	No	1
7. If you could live where you wanted, where would you live?	"Here" is the only +	
8. I sometimes worry so much that I can't sleep	No	1
	Yes	0
9. As I get older, things are better, worse, or the same as I thought they would be	Better	1
	Worse	0
	Same	0
10. I sometimes feel that life isn't worth living	Yes	0
	No	1
11. I am as happy now as I was when I was younger	Yes	1
	No	0
12. I have a lot to be sad about	No	1
	Yes	0
13. People had it better in the old days	Yes	0
	No	1
14. I am afraid of a lot of things	Yes	0
	No	1
15. I get mad more than I used to	No	1
	Yes	0
16. Life is hard for me most of the time	Yes	0
	No	1
17. How satisfied are you with your life today?	Not satisfied	0
	Satisfied	1
18. I take things hard	No	1
	Yes	0
19. A person has to live for today and not worry about tomorrow	No	0
	Yes	1
20. My health is the same, better, or worse than most people my age	Better	1
	Same	1
	Worse	0
21. I get upset easily	No	1
	Yes	0

aspects of psychiatric symptomatology, thinking, and social behavior are covered in this schedule. With appropriate training it may be completed by observers who are not psychiatrists.* One of the better ward behavior rating scales, the Stockton Rating Scale, was devised by Meer and Baker expressly for the geriatric patient.[26] In addition to the usual items dealing with deficits in physical self-maintenance, the 33 items contain scales for apathy, communication failure, and socially irritating behavior. However, in consideration of the fact that instrument development in this area is in such an early stage, it may be preferable to rely on the usual clinical psychiatric evaluation if a general noninstitutional assessment of psychiatric status is desired.

Comment

The availability of specific measures of functioning in these different areas makes it relatively easy to get a picture of how a specific older person compares with other elderly people. The entire set of functions might not necessarily have to be tested in order to arrive at some treatment-relevant conclusions. In any case, the procedures would act as a skeleton for the total clinical assessment. None of them is precise enough to be used rigidly, with cut-off points for decision-making. However, clinical decisions made with the assistance of these formal devices may be a distinct improvement over those made solely on the basis of "clinical feel."

REFERENCES

1. Lawton, M. P.: Assessing the competence of older people, in Kent, D., Kastenbaum, R. and Sherwood, S. (Eds.): Research, Planning, and Action for the Elderly. New York, Behavioral Publications (in press).
2. Lawton, M. P.: Problems in functional assessment. Paper presented at the Annual Meeting of the Gerontological Society, Denver, Colorado. November 1968.
3. Lawton, M. P.; Ward, M., and Yaffe, S.: Indices of health in an aging population, J. Gerontol. 22:334, 1967.
4. Wyler, A. R.; Masuda, M., and Holmes, T. H.: Seriousness of illness rating scale, J. Psychosom. Res. 11:363, 1968.
5. Burack, B.: Interdisciplinary classification for the aged, J. Chron. Dis. 18:1059, 1965.
6. Maddox, G.: Self-assessment of health status, J. Chron. Dis. 17:449, 1964.
7. Sokolow, J.; Silson, J.; Taylor, E.; Anderson, E., and Rusk, H.: A new approach to the objective evaluation of physical disability, J. Chron. Dis. 15:105, 1962.
8. Waldman, A., and Fryman, E.: Classification in homes for the aged, in Shore, H. and Leeds, M. (Eds.): Geriatric Institutional Management. New York, Putnam, 1964, pp. 131-135.
9. Katz, S.; Downs, T. D.; Cash, H. R., and Grotz, R. C.: Progress in development of the index of ADL, Gerontologist 10:20, 1970 (Part I).
10. Lowenthal, M. F.: Lives in Distress. New York, Basic Books, 1964.
11. Lawton, M. P., and Brody, E.: Assessment of older people: self-maintaining and instrumental activities of daily living, Gerontologist 9:179, 1969.

*Information on Mental Status Schedule forms, administration, and scoring may be obtained from Biometrics Research, 722 W. 168 St., New York, N. Y. 10032.

12. Kahn, R. L.; Pollack, M., and Goldfarb, A. I.: Factors related to individual differences in mental status of institutionalized aged. New York State Department of Mental Hygiene, Office for Aging. (Mimeo report, undated.)
13. Lawton, M. P.: Schizophrenia forty-five years later, J. Genet. Psychol. (in press).
14. Farina, A.; Arenberg, D., and Guskin, S.: A scale for measuring minimal social behavior, J. Consult. Psychol. **21**:265, 1957.
15. Cavan R. S.; Burgess, E. W.; Havighurst, R. J., and Goldhamer, H.: Personal Adjustment in Old Age. Chicago, Science Research Associates, 1949.
16. Havighurst, R.: The social competence of middle-aged people, Genet. Psychol. Monogr. **56**:297, 1957.
17. Havighurst, R. J.; Munnichs, J. M. A.; Neugarten, B. L., and Thomae, H.: Adjustment to Retirement—A Cross-National Study. New York, Humanities Press, 1969.
18. Rosow, I.: Adjustment of the normal aged, in Williams, R. H., Tibbitts, C. and Donahue, W. (Eds.): Processes of Aging, Volume II. New York, Atherton, 1963, pp. 195-223.
19. Havighurst, R.: Successful aging, in Williams, R. H., Tibbitts, C. and Donahue, W. (Eds.): Processes of Aging, Volume I. New York, Atherton, 1963, pp. 299-320.
20. Lawton, M. P.: The dimensions of morale, in Kent, D., Kastenbaum, R. and Sherwood, S. (Eds.): Research, Planning, and Action for the Elderly. New York, Behavioral Publications (in press).
21. Kutner, B.; Fanshel, D.; Togo, A. M., and Langner, T. S.: Five Hundred Over Sixty. New York, Russell Sage Foundation, 1956.
22. Neugarten, B. L.; Havighurst, R. J., and Tobin, S. S.: The measurement of life satisfaction, J. Gerontol. **16**:134, 1961.
23. Cumming, E., and Henry, W.: Growing Old. New York, Basic Books, 1961.
24. Wood, V.; Wylie, M. L., and Sheafor, B.: An analysis of a short self-report measure of life satisfaction: correlation with rater judgments, J. Gerontol. **24**:465, 1969.
25. Spitzer, R. L.; Burdock, E. I.; Endicott, J.; Cohen, G. M.; Bennett, R., and Weinstock, C.: Mental Status Schedule, Geriatric Supplement. Biometrics Research, New York State Department of Mental Hygiene, New York City, 1966.
26. Meer, B., and Baker, J. A.: The Stockton Geriatric Rating Scale, J. Gerontol. **21**:392, 1966.

6 The design of supportive environments for the life-span*

WALTER M. BEATTIE, Jr., M.A.**

. . . Knowledge will be a safe weapon only if it is linked to a deeply rooted conviction that organizations are made for men and not men for organizations.

The whole purpose of such knowledge is to design environments conducive to individual fulfillment . . . (Gardner, 1963)

The above quotation by John Gardner suggests not only a philosophical stance on the uses of knowledge for the achievement of human purposes, but equally a view of environment design predicated upon human goals and social values. The question must be posed as to whether or not the design of environments properly begins with technology and physical arrangements to which man must adapt. It is the thesis of this paper that the beginning point of environmental design is man, his individual and social aspirations throughout the life-span. Such design must be predicated on a developmental view of man and provide a range of choices which support self-actualization and determination at each stage associated with the process of aging.

We live, especially those of us in Western Societies, more and more in so-called planned urban environments. New towns, experimental cities, and model cities within older communities are being designed and constructed at an ever increasing rate. Exciting technologies and innovations abound. Their relevance and usefulness in supporting the functional capacities and needs of man

Reproduced from The Gerontologist **10:** 190-193, Autumn, 1970. Part I.
*Invited paper presented at the Symposium for Social Planning and the Physical Environment, 8th International Congress on Gerontology, Washington, DC, Aug. 28, 1969
**Dean and Professor, School of Social Work, Syracuse University, Syracuse.

may be questioned. To date, much of the design of physical environments negate the capacities of individuals, particularly those in the latter-third of the life-span, to achieve personal and societal goals. It is suggested that a central purpose of environmental design is to create a set of physical, psychological, and social arrangements which support the functional capacities* of the individual and his group associations.

The concept of design, and indeed that of social planning, which is the theme of this symposium, *is to provide a structured approach to the achievement of desired goals.* It is based upon the view that certain factors or conditions can be manipulated (the means) to achieve stated ends. Aging, if viewed from a developmental perspective as encompassing the life-span, becomes a significant and central view, if the purpose of environmental design is to manipulate the human habitat to promote the achievement of the human potential at each stage of growth, maturation, and change. Kastenbaum (1968) has pointed out that

> Perhaps the most significant problem . . . is to avoid erroneously attributing aging of behavior to intrinsic developmental changes, where, in fact, there are other personal and environmental factors involved which could be manipulated if correctly identified.

Likewise, Duncan (1968) has stated:

> . . . Two very general conceptual schemes have evolved which provide a suitable framework for structuring our thoughts and studies on aging. One of these is developmental; the other is ecological. These two approaches are complementary. We must consider the effect of intrinsic and environmental factors on human development and aging. . . .
> . . . We will profit today if we take an extremely broad approach to the aging individual and all the environmental variables that impinge upon him.

Much as Duncan points to developmental and ecological conceptual schema "for structuring thoughts and studies on aging," the design of environments must also be so structured. We can view the human environment as a set of interdependent physical, psychological, and social arrangements which can negate or support the functional capacities of the individual and his group associations. The goal of sound social planning must be that of achieving an environment to support rather than negate such capacities.

Man lives in a world of physical objects as well as in a defined territory under specified climatic conditions. This is true for all members of the animal kingdom. However, for man, the objective of controlling and bending the environment through technology has permitted increasing freedom from the limiting and maladaptive aspects of that environment. It has also led to cultural determinants which may restrict as well as free man.

---

*By functional capacity is meant those physiological, intellectual, and emotional characteristics of the individual which are expressed in behavior or which have potential for such expression.

For example, a critical requirement for all men is locomotion and mobility. The inventions of the automobile and airplane have freed man from a specific locale. Such inventions, however, influence more than transportation and have become basic determinants in the design of urban communities. They create vast and predictable movements of populations on a daily as well as seasonal basis. However, their access and use may be limited and not appropriate to all stages of the life-span. For the very aged they may be restrictive.

The physical design of environments, such as the location and construction of highways, airports, parking lots, etc., may become barriers to the accessibility and utilization of basic survival requirements of man. Physical space, open space, and the aesthetics of a territory, within a community, a neighborhood, or residential environment—independent or congregate—may support or negate functional capacity.

Man's environment is also psychological (Hall, 1959, 1966). Schooler (1969) suggests research approaches which relate environmental factors to psychological and adjustment measures. He concludes

> ... That the environment is not simply the screen against which the dynamics of life are enacted, but rather the matrix not only from which, but within which, the quality of certain life processes are determined.

This is not to posit a view of environmental determinism of behavior. It is to underscore the interdependence of the psychological with the physical environment. The psychological environment must be a concern of social planning. It includes perceptions and meanings regarding the physical environment and its objects, including what has been called psychological space. Further, it encompasses the interrelationships of perceptual, cognitive, and affective states of the individual to the physical and interpersonal environments with which he interacts. It is posited that social planning must include psychological environmental considerations.

Finally, and here there is a paucity of research data, is the dimension of the social environment. It includes cultural identities, group interactions, and meanings—past, present, and future. Here the concept of social space, which must be afforded man in his group associations, is essential. Too often social planning has stressed the role and uses of health and social services to support function without viewing the importance of designing environments which strengthen primary and secondary group associations and social institutional arrangements. It is suggested that the design of environments which permit adaptation and responsiveness of human institutions and social arrangements to the special requirements of the individual may be more essential than the artifact of social services, which tend, all too often, to be organized around the needs and constraints of the provider rather than the goals and requirements of the consumer.

The concept of supportive environments—physical, psychological, and social—which are organized and oriented toward the promotion of functional capacities—biological/physiological and psychological/social—of the individual to promote maximum realization of potential self-determination is essential. Critical is the need to formulate ways of assessing functional capacities and the development of criteria for such assessment.* Pioneering efforts in this direction hopefully will lead to predictive instruments based upon verifiable criteria. Data must be assembled and knowledge constructed to encompass functional capacities at each stage of the life-span.

A central premise of environmental design is that man is capable of rational thought and that he can bring his creativity to bear upon the design of his environment.† In discussing the roles of social planning in environmental design it is imperative that they not be viewed in the light of past tradition, purposes, and functions, but rather be redefined around human expectations and social realities which can be envisioned for man in the 21st century. If we agree with the 18th century poet and philosopher, Alexander Pope, that "man is the measure of all things," then the starting place in the design of environments must begin with man, our knowledge about him, and from this evolve a social design.

Although the social and behavioral sciences compared with the physical and biological sciences are still in their infancy, we are beginning to amass some knowledge which views man in his developmental aspects—biological, psychological, and sociological—from earliest infancy through old age. It is envisioned that a social design can be realistically developed based upon our knowledge of such developmental and aging processes. This would mean a drawing together of knowledge concerning the common and basic needs for the early infant, the preschool child, the young school child, the preadolescent child, the adolescent, the young adult, those in their early maturity, those in late maturity, and those in their aged or later years.

If one of the characteristics as one moves through time and the developmental stages of adulthood, maturity, and old age is greater flexibility in the uses of time, with less emphasis on work-productivity and family responsibilities, then we begin to perceive the requirement of a physical-psychological social environment which supports choice for the individual and gives meaning to his uses of time.

Perhaps an example is in order here. Because of our more traditional emphasis and value orientations toward work and productivity, societal institutions such as education have been perceived primarily as preparing individuals for early adulthood economic roles as producers. In the United States the community institution of the public school has been organized to socialize

---

*The difficulty of the task is pointed up in the Final Report, Functional Appraisal of Aging Individuals. (Gerontological Society, 1968.)

†The views for the remainder of this paper are adapted from preliminary statements developed by the author for the Minnesota Experimental City.

the child for early adulthood responsibilities in the home and at work. The concept of the public school is one that is open from 8 a.m. to 5 p.m., with noon luncheon programs and minimal recreational facilities. Increasingly, due to a number of pressing social issues, concepts of bussing and the construction of campus-planned facilities which would negate neighborhood-based schools have come into being. The physical design and spatial location of schools for the next third of the century are being determined without looking at the broader role of education and the possible uses of time for the entire life-span.

If we recognize the need for human association, creative growth, new experiences, information exchange, etc.—at all stages of life—we might begin to reconceptualize the role and functions of education in community life. What is argued is that a developmental-aging perspective as the conceptual base for social planning will lead to new institutional forms and ecological arrangements in the physical design of communities—including housing, institutional, and congregate care facilities.

If we so perceive the functions of education to relate to the requirements of the human condition for the adult and aging years, and as having broader cultural and recreational purposes in addition to occupational preparation, then such a facility might be designed to be open from 8 a.m. to midnight, expand its food service facilities into the evening hours, and be accessible to *all* the generations—in family groups and as individuals. Such a public educational facility could offer a range of activities and pursuits to support more flexible "life-styles" and preferences for each developmental stage—in concert or individually.

Other human and social institutional forms could be so assessed, with new social and physical designs emerging. Time does not permit their explication. Suffice it to say that new conceptualizations of neighborhoods, accessibility, availability, and acceptability of resources, and the roles of consumers and providers should emerge. Of particular interest should be new designs of social utilities which give new form and viability to the more traditional view of public and private sectors of responsibility.

It is proposed that an examination be carried out to identify from existing research what is common to all regardless of age-related changes; what is unique, based upon common characteristics and needs at specific developmental and aging periods; what constitutes common and unique characteristics, such as social economic status, racial characteristics and ethnic identity and so forth; and, what value orientations should be stressed to support and permit the fulfillment of creative, renewing, and self-mastery needs of the individual at all stages of the life-span and for all sectors of the community. Such a design could, it is envisioned, if developed along an age-related continuum, permit social interaction within age-specific groups as well as age-intergeneration groups and would support our emerging knowledge of basic demographic and ecological changes occuring with urbanization. In other words, the design of the city would support rather than negate the concept of intergenerational family relationships. It would permit greater viability as to changing concepts of the meaningful use of time by interrelating family and living arrangements with occupational and leisure pursuits, cultural and spiritual self-renewing activities, and family interdependence.

Inherent throughout such a construct is the view that social planning as related to physical design must emphasize the essential requirement of choice. Such choice must be related to the capabilities of environments in providing alternatives in decision-making and self-determination by the individual and his family. Again, I would emphasize the importance of viewing human development and aging within the context of the family. The social milieu and physical environment—whether within the macrocosm of the community or the microcosm of the home or congregate care facility—must be designed to assure a range of alternatives which enable maximum growth and use of functional capacities. Admittedly this is a value-loaded orientation. Values are, in my judgment, central to the basic issues of our urban dilemmas. Those which focus on the unique requirements and potentials of the individual as he moves in time (the life-span) and space, provide new ecological constructs for urban and physical design.

The above is predicated upon a view of a society which is continually expanding in population, where the special needs of the very young and the very old will increase (by 1975 it is predicted that approximately one-half of the population of the United States will be under 18 or over 65 years of age), where productivity in the economic sense will be increasingly relegated to technological innovations requiring fewer man hours, and where the issue of the meaningful use of time, including leisure time will not be restricted to the concept of 18th century economic man. It suggests that human institutions must have as their goals the support of the individual in achieving the optimum functioning of which he is capable while at the same time providing protection and security. It further will emphasize new dimensions of human interdependence through a realignment of the institutions of the family, the economic, the social, and the political to assure the individual alternatives and choices while at the same time participation in a set of human relationships.

It is, therefore, suggested that there is need for precise definitions of common and divergent human needs and characteristics as related to age, sex, marital status, and so forth. There is further need to develop criteria for functional assessments at each stage of the life-span as well as the role of varying environmental characteristics to support a variety of levels of function. The place of work, play, and family relations will have to be critically redesigned ecologically, and the aesthetic dimensions of man and his spiritual needs will be met through new approaches to physical, social, and psychological experiences.

A further dimension will be a redefinition of territory and mobility, again predicated upon the above concepts. It is envisioned, however, that these concepts can be defined only after the preceding have been clarified. The technology to create the physical dimensions of the city, it is argued, must follow such a concept of social design which emphasizes developmental dimensions of the life-span. Without such a construct it will be impossible to support the integrity and individuality of the human personality.

The above, therefore, is not a social-problem orientation toward the chaos of our modern urban centers, but rather it views as central to social planning of the physical environment the development of new conceptual frameworks which may serve as models for continuous experimentation. They may provide fundamental solutions to problems which now abound in our urban centers, including those associated with aging.

REFERENCES

Duncan, L. E., Jr. Ecology and aging. Gerontologist, 1968, **8,** 80-83.

Gardner, J. W. Self-renewal. New York: Harper & Row, 1963.

Gerontological Society. Final report (Contract No. PH 110-100), Functional appraisal of aging individuals, 1968.

Hall, E. T. The silent language. New York: Doubleday, 1959.

Hall, E. T. The hidden dimension. New York: Doubleday, 1966.

Kastenbaum, R. Perspectives on the development and modification of behavior in the aged: A developmental-field perspective. Gerontologist, 1968, **8,** 280-283.

Schooler, K. K. The relationship between social interaction and morale in the elderly as a function of environmental characteristics. Gerontologist, 1969, **9,** 25-29.

The effects of aging on activities and attitudes*

ERDMAN B. PALMORE, Ph.D.**

[Does aging reduce activities and attitudes? Most cross-sectional surveys agree that it does, but recent longitudinal evidence tends to question the extent of this reduction. Are decreases in activities related to decreases in satisfaction? Disengagement theory maintains that high satisfaction in aging results from acceptance of the "inevitable" reduction in interaction, while "activity theory" maintains that reduction in activity results in reduction of satisfaction. Is there a persistence of life style among the aged? There is evidence that, regardless of the average effects of aging, individual persons tend to maintain relatively high or relatively low levels of activity and satisfaction during their later years. Does aging increase homogeneity or differentiation? Again, theories have been advanced supporting both positions.]

Such questions and theories have fascinated social gerontologists for at least the two decades since the Chicago group developed their Activity and Attitude Inventory (Cavan, Burgess, Havighurst, & Goldhamer, 1949). A major reason for the uncertain answers and conflicting theories is that usually cross-sectional data were used even though these questions deal with change over time. It was not until 1963 that longitudinal data were first presented in an attempt to clarify these uncertainties (Maddox, 1963). The present paper discusses new longitudinal findings relevant to these questions from data that now cover a ten-year period of tests and retests.

Reproduced from The Gerontologist 8:259-263, Winter, 1968.
*The research on which this paper is based was supported in part by Grant HD-00668, National Institute of Child Health and Human Development, USPHS. The computations involved were carried out in the Duke University Computing Laboratory, which is supported in part by the National Science Foundation. Programming for the computations was done by Mrs. Nancy Watson.
**Center for the Study of Aging and Human Development, Duke University, Durham, N.C. 27706.

61

Methods

One hundred twenty-seven (out of 256) volunteer participants in a longitudinal, interdisciplinary study of aging were examined and interviewed the first time during 1955-1959 and were reinterviewed at approximately three-year intervals so that they had completed four waves of interviews by 1966-1967.* When interviewed the fourth time, they ranged in age from 70 to 93 with a mean age of 78. Fifty-one were men and 76 were women. There was less than one year's difference between the mean age for men and the mean age for women. All were ambulatory, noninstitutionalized residents of the central North Carolina area. The initial panel of 256 persons did not consitute a random sample of Durham residents, but were chosen from a larger number of volunteers so that their sex, racial, and occupational distribution approximated that of the area. Nevertheless, analysis of selection and attrition factors indicates that the panelists were a social, psychological, and physical elite among the aged and became more so through time (Maddox, 1962). However, since longitudinal analysis uses each S as his own control and examines changes over time rather than comparing younger with older Ss, the degree to which the sample of an age category represents the universe of an age category is a less critical issue than in cross-sectional studies.

We need not discuss here the various advantages of longitudinal analysis for studying aging, such as its greater sensitivity and its ability to measure change directly rather than inferentially (Goldfarb, 1960; Maddox, 1965), but we might point out one advantage of repeated measurements that has not been widely recognized. This is the ability to use consistency as a test of reliable and significant change when one has three or more repeated measurements on the same sample. When a change is observed between two points in time, there is always the possibility that this change might be due to temporary or chance fluctuations. But when the same change is observed between the second and third points in time, our confidence in the reliability and significance of this change can be greatly increased because the probability of two such changes occurring by chance is much smaller. Thus, in the present discussion we shall focus on consistent changes (or lack of consistency) as well as on the statistically significant changes.

The Inventory of Activity and Attitudes questions were read to the Ss by a social worker as part of a longer social history. The Activity Inventory consists of 20 questions dealing with five areas of activities (about four questions for each area): health (physical capacity to act); family and friends (frequency of contacts); leisure (ways of spending time, hobbies, reading, organizations); economic (amount of work or housework and lack of economic restrictions on activity); and religious activity (attendance at religious services, listening to them

---

*A few Ss missed the second or third wave of interviews but all 127 returned for the fourth wave.

on radio or TV, reading religious literature).* Each sub-score could range from zero to ten with the higher scores indicating more activity. The total activity score is the sum of the sub-scores in these five areas (total range: 0-50).

The Attitude Inventory consists of 56 agree-disagree items about the S's satisfaction with eight areas of his life (seven items in each area): health, friends, work, economic security, religion, usefulness, family, and general happiness.† The score in each area could range from zero to six (one item of the seven is neutral in the scoring) with the higher scores indicating more satisfaction. The total attitude score is the sum of the scores in these eight areas (total range: 0-48). Further discussion of the development, purpose, scoring, reliability, and validity of these inventories may be found in Cavan et al. (1949) and Havighurst (1951). These inventories have been used in more than 20 different studies and the results show a relatively high degree of reliability and validity.

As a check on the Inventory of Activity and Attitudes, the social worker interviewing the Ss used the Cavan Adjustment Rating Scale to give her estimation of the Ss' activities and attitudes (Havighurst & Albrecht, 1953). In general, the results from these scales were similar to those from the Activity and Attitude Inventory.

Some may question the appropriateness of comparing mean scores and correlations on the grounds that such analysis assumes equal intervals in the scales even though we are not sure this assumption is justified. However, several statisticians have recently pointed out that treating ordinal scales as equal-interval scales (1) involves assumptions that may be no more misleading than the use of arbitrary cutpoints that obscure differences in amount of variation (Blalock, 1961); (2) has been useful in developing more accurate measurements and theory in most sciences (Burke, 1963); (3) usually involves relatively little error (Labovitz, 1967); and in general allows much more powerful and sensitive analysis. Since we are interested primarily in direction of change and relative changes rather than absolute amounts of change, this type of analysis seems worth the risk of assuming equal intervals.

Results

Small reductions. The men had almost no over-all reduction over the ten years in either activities or attitudes (Tables 1 and 2). The women had significant but quite small (less than 7%) reductions in both activities and attitudes. This lack of substantial reduction in activities is contrary to disengagement theory

---

*Typical questions: How many days did you spend in bed last year? How often do you see some of your family or close relatives? How many club meetings do you usually attend each month? Are you working now (full-time, part-time, or not working)? How often do you attend religious services?

†Typical items: I feel just miserable most of the time. I have all the good friends anyone could wish. I am satisfied with the work I now do. I am just able to make ends meet. Religion is a great comfort to me. My life is meaningless now. I am perfectly satisfied with the way my family treats me. My life is full of worry.

Table 1. Mean activity scores at four points in time

Activities	Time 1	Time 2	Time 3	Time 4
Men:				
Health	2.4	3.9*	3.1	2.6
Family and friends	6.8	7.5	6.8	6.9
Leisure	6.9	5.8*	5.7*	5.6*
Economic	4.8	4.9	5.3	6.0
Religious	6.3	6.1	5.5	6.0
Total	27.2	28.2	26.4	27.1
Women:				
Health	2.5	3.2	2.6	2.5
Family and friends	5.9	6.1	5.5	5.3*
Leisure	7.7	7.2	6.6*	6.3*
Economic	7.4	7.5	8.1	8.4*
Religious	6.7	7.1	6.4	6.7
Total	30.2	31.1	29.2*	29.2*

*Difference between this score and score at Time 1 is significant at .01 level according to the *t*-test for paired observations.

Table 2. Mean attitude scores at four points in time

Attitudes	Time 1	Time 2	Time 3	Time 4
Men:				
Health	3.8	3.7	4.1	3.5
Friends	4.6	4.4	4.3	4.2
Work	3.7	3.6	3.8	3.4
Economic security	3.3	3.6	4.0*	3.7
Religion	5.2	5.3	5.3	5.5*
Usefulness	4.3	4.3	4.3	4.0
Family	4.9	4.6	4.9	5.0
Happiness	4.3	4.4	3.6*	4.1
Total	34.1	33.9	34.3	33.4
Women:				
Health	4.0	3.8	3.7	3.6*
Friends	4.5	4.4	4.5	4.3
Work	3.9	3.8	3.7	3.5*
Economic security	3.8	3.9	4.0*	4.0*
Religion	5.5	5.6	5.7*	5.6
Usefulness	4.6	4.3	4.4	4.1*
Family	4.7	4.8	4.9	4.8
Happiness	4.2	4.1	3.6*	3.6*
Total	35.2	34.7	34.5*	33.5*

*Difference between this score and score at Time 1 is significant at .01 level according to the *t*-test for paired observations.

Table 3. Correlations (r) of changes in activities with changes in total attitudes (Time 1 to Time 4)

Activity	Men	Women
Health	.07	.09
Family and friends	.12	.27*
Leisure	.22	.10
Economic	.36*	.30*
Religious	.26	.13
Total activity	.42*	.40*

*The probability of this correlation occurring by chance is less than .01.

which asserts that marked withdrawal from activities is the modal pattern in aging (Cumming & Henry, 1961). It is also contrary to the findings of most cross-sectional surveys (for example, Havighurst & Albrecht, 1953) and contrary to the commonly held assumption that most people become less active as they age. On the other hand, it is consistent with previous longitudinal findings from this panel (Maddox, 1963) (Table 3).

There are two plausible explanations for this apparent contradictions. While the aged may disengage or reduce activities in *some* areas such as belonging to organizations and attending meetings (as shown by the declining leisure activities scores) or retiring from work (most of our panel was already retired), they may compensate by increasing activities in other areas such as contacts with family and friends or reading religious literature. Or a temporary decrease may be compensated for by a subsequent increase. Or some may reduce while others increase. The net effect would then be little or no change in the average total activities score. Second, this panel represents those relatively healthy aged who were community residents and who survived for over ten years from the first wave to their fourth wave, "ripe old age," of 70 to 93. It may be that the relatively healthy aged do maintain a fairly stable plateau of activity up until just before death and that it is only the ill or disabled aged who pull the average activity level down in cross-sectional studies. The cross-sectional association of poor health and low activity is well established (Jeffers & Nichols, 1961; Havighurst & Albrecht, 1953). The same explanations would apply to the mixed changes in attitudes which show some increases, some decreases, and no significant net decrease in total attitudes among men.

It is unlikely that this pattern of small or insignificant decreases could be attributed to unreliability in the tests, because the reliability of these tests has been demonstrated elsewhere and is confirmed in this study by the moderately high correlations of earlier scores with later scores (Table 4).

The fact that women had larger and more consistent decreases in both activities and attitudes seems to indicate that aging produces greater net changes

Table 4. Correlations (r) of earlier score with later score for total activities and total attitudes

Variable	Time 1 with Time 2	Time 2 with Time 3	Time 3 with Time 4	Time 1 with Time 4
Men:				
Total activities	.57	.57	.46	.27
Total attitudes	.74	.73	.71	.65
Women:				
Total activities	.75	.65	.74	.60
Total attitudes	.67	.66	.79	.56

for women than men, at least in this age range. This may be related to the fact that most of the men had already retired before the beginning of this study and thus did not have to adjust to that change in status during the course of the study. Indeed, their increasing economic activity scores indicate that many men went back to work or increased their work during the study.

The small but significant increases of interest in religion, despite no increase in religious activities, confirm the findings of the cross-sectional studies (Moberg, 1965). This has been related to approaching death and increasing concern with after-life. However, Havighurst (1951) found that religious attitudes had practically no correlations with the total scores nor with the other sub-scores. He suggested that, since the religious items seemed to be measuring a different kind of dimension from the rest of the attitude scale, they should not be included in the total score. We also found that the religious attitude scores had almost no correlation with the total attitude score at any point in time (most of the correlations were less than .15) and that many of the correlations with the other sub-scores were even negative. We agree with Havighurst that the religion items should be dropped or considered separately from the rest of the attitude scale.

Activity correlates with attitudes. Changes in total activities were significantly and positively correlated with changes in total attitudes (Table 3). This means that those who reduced their activities as they aged tended to suffer reduction in over-all satisfaction, and, conversely, those who increased activities tended to enjoy an increase in satisfaction. This finding is contrary to what might be predicted from disengagement theory which asserts that disengagement is associated with the maintenance of high morale (Cumming & Henry, 1961). Even though disengagement is more than reduced activity, and morale is not exactly equivalent to our measure of satisfaction, it is fair to say that disengagement theory would probably predict no association or a negative association between changes in activity and changes in attitudes. That is, when activities decrease, attitudes should remain high or even increase, rather than decline as in our study.

This positive correlation of activity with attitudes supports rather the activity theory of aging which has been stated as the "American formula for happiness in old age . . . keep active" (Havighurst & Albrecht, 1953). This theory is favored by most of the practical workers in the field of gerontology:

> They believe that people should maintain the activities and attitudes of middle age as long as possible and then find substitutes for the activities which they must give up—substitutes for work when they are forced to retire; substitutes for clubs and associations which they must give up; substitutes for friends and loved ones whom they lose by death (Havighurst, 1961).

It may well be that disengagement theory is applicable to some and the activity theory is applicable to others; that some find most satisfaction in disengaging and others find most satisfaction in remaining active. But apparently in our panel the activity theory was most applicable to most of the participants.

Among the specific activities related to attitudes, change in economic activities were the most closely related to changes in total attitudes. This is congruent with Kutner's (1956) finding that having a job is more closely associated with high morale than is keeping busy with recreational activities. However, because the economic activities sub-scale contains an item on the restrictions on activities resulting from lower income we cannot be sure at this point whether it is the change in job status or change in income or both that account for the association with attitudes.

Changes in health had almost no association with changes in total attitudes. This is surprising in view of the substantial associations between health and activity on the one hand and between activity and attitudes on the other. Perhaps this indicates that unless health changes activity, there is little effect on attitudes.

Persistence of life style. There is a clear tendency for aged people to persist with the same relative levels of activities and attitudes as they grow older. Most of the correlations of earlier scores with scores three years later were .57 or higher; half were over .70 (Table 4). This means that over half of the variance in later scores can be accounted for by the earlier scores in the majority of comparisons. Correlations between scores at Time 1 with scores at Time 4 (ten years later) were much lower because of the greater time lapse which made possible a greater number of events that could change the relative levels of activity and attitudes.

This persistence in scores over three-year periods, and even over the entire ten years, indicates both that the inventories are fairly reliable and that patterns of behavior and attitudes among the aged tend to be fairly stable over long periods of time. This also supports the results of a different type of persistence analysis (Maddox, 1966).

However, the correlations do not show consistent trends toward increasing persistence in the later intervals. The men's correlations actually decline

Table 5. Standard deviations for activity and attitude scores at four points in time

Variables	Time 1	Time 2	Time 3	Time 4
Men:				
Total activities S. D.	6.2	6.5	6.1	5.4
Total attitudes S. D.	4.9	5.3	5.3	5.7
Women:				
Total activities S. D.	5.8	6.3	6.6	5.7
Total attitudes S. D.	5.5	5.5	5.5	5.8

somewhat in the third interval. Thus, the idea that the aged become increasingly rigid and "set in their ways" is not supported by this data.

Increasing homogeneity. The standard deviations show no consistent trend toward either increasing homogeneity or differentiation (Table 5). The women's standard deviations remained about the same while the men's decreased in activities but increased in attitudes. However, there was a generally consistent decrease in differences between the mean scores for men and women (Tables 1 and 2). There is practically no difference left between men and women in their total attitude scores by Time 3 and 4.

Thus, these data do not support the ideas that the aged become more differentiated in their behavior or attitudes (Havighurst, 1957) or that the "sexes become increasingly divergent with age" (Neugarten, 1964). On the contrary, the decrease in differences between men and women is consistent with Cameron's (1968) recent finding of converging interests between aged men and women.

Summary

Changes in activities and attitudes over a ten-year period among 127 panelists in a longitudinal study of aging were assessed by use of the Chicago Inventory of Activity and Attitudes. There was no significant over-all decrease in activities or attitudes among men and only small over-all decreases among women. This was interpreted as evidence contrary to the findings of most cross-sectional surveys and the commonly held assumption that most people become less active as they age. It was suggested that normal aging persons tend to compensate for reductions in some activities or attitudes by increases in others, or to compensate reductions at one point in time with increases at other times. The greater decreases among women seem to indicate that at this stage in life aging causes more over-all changes among women than men.

Changes in activities were positively correlated with changes in attitudes so that reductions in activity were associated with decreases in satisfaction. This was interpreted as contrary to disengagement theory but supportive of activity theory: the "American formula for happiness in old age . . . keep active."

There was a strong tendency for the panelists to persist with the same over-all level of activities and attitudes over time, but there was no evidence that patterns of behavior or attitudes became increasingly rigid or differentiated. In fact, mean differences between men and women tended to disappear.

REFERENCES

Blalock, H. M.: Causal Inferences in Nonexperimental Research. Univ. N. C. Press, Chapel Hill, 1961.

Burke, C. J.: Measurement scales and statistical models. In: M. H. Marx (Editor), Theories in Contemporary Psychology. Macmillan Co., New York, 1963.

Cavan, R. S., E. W. Burgess, R. J. Havighurst, and H. Goldhamer: Personal Adjustment in Old Age. Science Research Associates, Chicago, 1949, 204 pp.

Cameron, P.: Masculinity-femininity in the aged. J. Geront., 10:63-65, 1968.

Cumming, E., and W. E. Henry: Growing Old. Basic Books, New York, 1961.

Goldfarb, N.: Longitudinal Statistical Analysis. Free Press, Glencoe, Ill., 1960.

Havighurst, R. J.: Validity of the Chicago Attitude Inventory as a measure of personal adjustment in old age. J. Abnorm. (Soc.) Psychol., 461:24-29, 1951.

Havighurst. R. J.: The social competence of middle-aged people. Genet. Psychol. Monogr., 56:297-375, 1957.

Havighurst, R. J.: Successful aging. Gerontologist, 1:4-7, 1961.

Havighurst, R. J., and R. Albrecht: Older People. Longmans, Green, New York, 1953.

Jeffers, F. C., and C. R. Nichols: The relationship of activities and attitudes to physical well-being in older people. J. Geront., 16:67-70, 1961.

Kleemeier, R. W.: Leisure and disengagement in retirement. Gerontologist, 4:180-184, 1964.

Kutner, B.: Five hundred over sixty. Russell Sage Foundation, New York, 1956.

Labovitz, S.: Some observations on measurement and statistics. Soc. Forces, 46:151-160, 1967.

Maddox, G.: A longitudinal, multidisciplinary study of human aging. Proc. Social Statistics Section, Amer. Stat. Ass., 280-285, 1962.

Maddox, G.: Activity and morale: a longitudinal study of selected elderly subjects. Soc. Forces, 42:195-204, 1963.

Maddox, G.: Fact and artifact: evidence bearing on disengagement theory from the Duke Geriatrics Project. Hum. Develop., 8:117-130, 1965.

Maddox, G.: Persistence of life style among the elderly. Proc. 7th Internat. Congr. Geront., Wien. Med. Akad., Wien, 1966.

Moberg, D. O.: Religiosity in old age, Gerontologist, 51:78-87, 1965.

Neugarten, B. L.: A developmental view of adult personality. In: J. E. Birren (Editor), Relations of Development and Aging. Charles C Thomas, Springfield, Ill., 1964.

The foreshortened life perspective

ROBERT KASTENBAUM, Ph.D.*

The elderly person is marked in more ways than one. His face, hands, and all those body parts which are significant in social communication have become unmistakably engraved with age. Before he speaks, he has already identified himself to others as a person who occupies an extreme position in the spectrum of life. Should his words and actions also betray those features we associate with advanced age, then we are further encouraged to mark him down as one who is strikingly different from ourselves.

He is also marked by numbers, of course. In the case of the elderly person, the statistics relentlessly intersect and pursue. Begin any place. Begin by tracing the declining function of this organ system or that one. Begin by measuring changes in the musculoskeletal system or the speed of central nervous system activity. Begin by locating the elderly person within the actuarial charts. Wherever we begin, it is clear that the numbers have a common bias; they are all against him.

These markings, however, do not tell the whole story. As a matter of fact, they provide only the background and props. It is true enough that any of us might contrive the story of any elderly person's life, based upon these externals. We could manufacture suppositions about what he is experiencing within these biological and statistical markings—how he regards the past, how he views the future, and all the rest. The pity of it is—we do this sort of thing much of the time, without realizing that what we are hearing is not his story, but merely the sound of our own voices. It is so easy to suppose that he feels the way we think we would feel if we were in his situation, or simply that he must feel the way we

Reproduced from Geriatrics, August, 1969, pp. 126-133.
*Professor of Psychology, Wayne State University, Detroit, Michigan.

think it proper for an elderly person to feel. Any time we begin with such a misstep we are likely to accumulate even further distortions. We are likely to generalize without correctives. We are likely to develop set ways of dealing with the way we think he is.

How does the elderly person actually view his own life? What is his perspective and how did he happen to develop it? What functions does it perform for him? In what ways might his perspective affect the course of his own life and the lives of others? Of his total life experiences—past, present, and potentially future—what has he included? What has he excluded? Has he settled upon this perspective as a fixed, permanent vantage point, or are other orientations to come? Most basically, has he managed to create a symbolic structure that comes to terms with his total existence at the very time that this existence itself has become so vulnerable?

To gain perspective on the life perspective of aged people, it might be helpful to back up all the way to infancy. Does the infant have a life perspective? Quite on the contrary—he is almost totally engrossed in life. He experiences the moment. He does not reexperience the past or preexperience the future, at least not in that sense which depends upon the development of symbolic structures. One of the most profound differences between infant and adult is the raw experiencing of the moment, an experiencing that lacks the protection afforded by perspective. Although this point may be an obvious one, it should be emphasized because it is important in a different light in the phenomenological world of the aged.

Very quickly, the infant comes to appreciate the difference between a presence and an absence. At first, this awareness does not distinguish between temporal and spatial dimensions. Either something (for example, smiling-mother-presenting-lunch) is both here-and-now or it is absent—totally absent. By contrast, the adult differentiates "absence" into several alternatives that have differential meanings to him: something exists now, but not here, in this space; or, something will be in this space at a later time; or something has been in this space, but at a previous time; or, again, something is neither here nor there, now, then, or ever.

Such distinctions, and many others that are crucial to the development of a life perspective, come later in life, but the first gropings toward a perspective begin in infancy. There is a clear directional movement. The infant becomes increasingly liberated from its biology, on the one side, and its immediate environment, on the other. The directional thrust is a general process that must be distinguished from what might be called the solidified achievements of human development. This is perhaps the most fundamental basis for challenging the notion that the aged person and the child have a great deal in common. Although certain similarities do exist, the fact remains that it is only the child who is being carried forward on the tide of psychobiological development. All of his behavior and experience is marked by the directional thrust.

The surge of general development continues with great vigor throughout the childhood years and is manifested in physical, social, and psychological changes. Although all of these developments contribute to the emergence of life perspectives, two of the most salient psychological discoveries that children make are:

1. *The discovery of futurity.* This discovery has several components. First, there is the discovery of future time in the sense that "when this moment is over, there will be some more time coming." Secondly, there is the discovery of future time as qualitatively different from any other kind of time—it is fresh, unused time that can bring forth new experiences and events. This discovery implies a dawning appreciation of possibility and uncertainty. Third, there is the discovery of world or objective future time. Implied in this discovery is the realization that one does not really possess magical control over the universe and cannot really "take time out." Additionally, this is one of the insights that prepares the child to appreciate that, for all his precious and self-evident individuality, he is simply one of many fellow creatures, all of whom dance (or drag) to the music of time.

2. *The discovery of mortality.* Some rudimentary appreciation of nonexistence may be achieved in early childhood, perhaps even before the conquest of language, but many additional years of development are required before the child can frame the concept of personal mortality. The proposition "I will die" is intimately related to the sense of futurity. It will be the continuing task of the adolescent and the adult to define the nature of this relationship for himself, to integrate the concepts of more time—fresh, new time—possibility, hope, trust, and uncertainty with the concepts of certain death.

The available evidence suggests that adolescence is usually the time during which the developing person begins seriously to create his life perspective. He has had many of the elements previously but now, for the first time, he also has the intellectual equipment to forge these elements into a perspective—and the psychosocial readiness to venture forth as his own self. Children have their notions—but it is adolescents who have ideologies. It is the transformation in thought that underlies the adolescent's changes in social behavior. He now can think about thought, compare ideal with reality, shatter the world as it is presented to him with his new tools of intellectual analysis, and at least try to put the pieces together again in a new and more satisfying manner.

Adolescence, then, is the time of life in which the act of trying to develop perspectives is dominant.

Other characteristics of adolescence are: First, the adolescent has a strong sense of moving into the future. This is not at all the same thing as planning for or visualizing the future; rather, it is a restless experiencing of the developmental current running within oneself.

Second, the adolescent typically projects his thought and feeling intensively into a fairly narrow sector of the future. It is the proximate future that counts, that decisive and eventful time which is just around the corner. Old age is so remote and unappealing a prospect that it hardly can be located at all on his projective charts.

Third, the adolescent often neglects the past, especially his personal past. Neglect may be too passive a word to describe this phenomenon. I have the impression that many adolescents are waging an active battle against the past, trying to put psychological distance between who-I-used-to-be and who-I'm-going-to-be.

Finally, there is the adolescent's way of coming to terms with finality. The prospect of death, like the prospect of aging, often is regarded as a notion that is so remote as to have no relevance to one's own life. Death is avoided, glossed over, kidded about, neutralized, and controlled by a cool, spectator type of orientation. This is on the level of what might be called self-conscious, socially communicated thought. However, more probing and indirect methods of assessment suggest that many adolescents are extremely concerned about death—both in the sense of attempting to fathom its nature and meaning and in the sense of confronting the actual prospect of their own demise. We are no longer surprised when we come across an adolescent whose behavior is influenced by the expectation that he may die at an early age. Indeed, a foreshortened life perspective is by no means the special prerogative of the aged person.

What happens to life perspective during the adult years? We know less about mature perspectives than any other sort, but I think the life perspective of a mature adult has the following characteristics:

It is, first of all, a genuine perspective. This means that the individual has been able to subdivide his life-space into multiple points which stretch away in both directions from the present moment. He is able to locate himself at any one of these points and utilize the other points to achieve the effect of perspective. He might, for example, evaluate the immediate situation in terms of its possible future consequences. A more complex perspective consists of evaluating the immediate situation in terms of both past and future circumstances. More complex still is the perspective in which the individual flexibly shifts the emphasis among past, present, and future standpoints, with all three orientations always involved but varying in relationship to each other. At one moment his pivotal concern may be with past events; thus he calls upon his immediate observations and future projections to provide a context of meaning around the past. At another moment he locates himself in the future and scans his past and present for what clues they can yield that would help him to comprehend his future self.

Upon closer inspection, his perspective will prove to be a structure that includes a variety of subperspectives. These might be visualized as operating in an umbrella type of arrangement. Opened slightly, the perspective system permits the individual to gain coverage of his proximate past and future. This could be called the yesterday-and-tomorrow framework. Opened more broadly, he now has perspective on a larger period of time, but this is still only a small range within his total life-span, where he has been and where he is going, relative to where he is now.

A mature use of the life perspective involves good judgment in deciding when it is appropriate to use a particular subperspective. It involves the ability to scan time in two distinctly different ways—the axiological and the probabilistic. In projecting future, for example, the individual identifies his hopes, fears, and values. This is the axiological orientation. But he also is capable of reading the future in a more objective style, trying to establish the most likely pattern of expectancies. The ability to sweep through time in both axiological and probabilistic styles seems to be one of the hallmarks of a mature life perspective that is maturely employed. Futhermore, there will be an optimal balance between perspectives-already-established and fresh perspective-seeking activities. A flexible life perspective makes it possible to identify and integrate the novel or unexpected event without scuttling the more enduring perspectivistic structure.

Just as important as the life perspective itself, however, is the ability to let go, to know when it is in one's best interests to become totally engrossed in a situation. All perspective and no engrossment makes for a barren, abstracted sort of life.

A mature life perspective is the type that permits a person to make constructive use of his past experiences without becoming enslaved to them and to confront his future, including the prospect of death, without capitulating in that direction either. Many people fail to develop a functional and versatile life perspective, however. In some cases we see a distorted or dysfunctional perspective; in other cases we are struck by the absence of perspective. These different psychological orientations cannot be expected to lead to the same situation when the individuals involved reach advanced age.

In exploring what has been learned and what has yet to be learned about life perspectives in the aged, we should examine the disengagement theory. This is not just a courtesy call to respect the contributions of Elaine Cumming and William E. Henry—it happens that the disengagement theory is one of the few conceptual orientations to make something of life perspectives in later adulthood. Everybody knows by now that the hypothetical process of disengagement involves a gradual and mutual withdrawal of the aging individual and his society. It is said to be an inevitable and normal developmental process. It is said to occur universally, or at least to occur universally under favorable conditions. Obviously, this is an important proposition. Is it also a true proposition? That is another question and one which would take us beyond the scope of this discussion.

But there is a relevant question here. How does the disengagement process itself get started? Cumming and Henry have suggested that disengagement begins with an event that takes place within ourselves, or more specifically, within our life perspectives. As we approach the later years of our lives we come to realize that our future is limited. There is not enough time left to do everything we had hoped and planned. Eventually we also realize that time is not only limited, but it is running out. Death comes into view as a salient prospect. Do Cumming and Henry mean that without this altered life perspective there would be no disengagement? They say: "It seems probable that disengagement would be resisted forever if there were no problem of the allocation of time and thus no anticipation of death. Questions of choice among alternative uses of time lead to curtailment of some activities. Questions of the inevitability of death lead to introspective reflections on the meaning of life."

Although this formulation emphasizes the importance of the individual's inner framework for organizing his experience and, in particular, the role of death anticipations, the formulation appears to be at variance with the facts. Although our knowledge of life perspectives is far from adequate, I believe that enough has been learned to indicate that the disengagement hypothesis has only limited application.

The disengagement hypothesis assumes that everybody has just about the same kind of perspective as they approach the later years of life. This generalization is not tenable. It is already clear that there are significant individual variations, even within particular subgroups in our own society. Some people, for example, never develop the complete umbrella of perspectives described earlier. They move through their life-span within a narrow shell of time, almost day-by-day. This kind of person does not wake up one morning and gasp, "My God, I have only a finite number of years ahead; I had best reallocate my time." The sound of distant drums never had much influence over him, and it may not get to him now, either. Many people in their seventh, eighth, and ninth decades maintain a well-entrenched narrow perspective.

By contrast, there are other people who have been brandishing a wide-open perspective umbrella ever since their youth. The use of time and the prospect of death are factors which have influenced their lives every step of the way. Such people confront different challenges than do those who may be first awakening to intimations of mortality, or those whose limited perspectives have been little influenced by the passing years.

Many people do not experience the altered outlook on time and death that Cumming and Henry proposed as the psychological trigger for disengagement, but even among those who do confront this prospect within their life perspectives, there are important variations. The disengagement theorists have stated that "The anticipation of death frees us from the obligation to participate in the ongoing stream of life. If there is only a little time left, there is no point in planning for a future and no point in putting off today's gratification."

On the contrary, many people intensify their participation in life in order to obtain the greatest possible yield from the time remaining to them. This orientation can persist well beyond the sixth and seventh decades. In studying the psychology of dying and death within a population of very aged patients in a geriatric hospital, we have encountered many who came to terms with approaching death by investing themselves solidly in the network of interpersonal life.

Furthermore, there is reason to believe that the aged person who does clamber out of "the ongoing stream of life" may be doing so for a different reason. Our research interviews suggest that in many cases the individual is not gracefully disengaging to enjoy today's gratification because the future is too short to support long-range plans. Rather, he is more likely to feel that he is no longer capable of making good use even of the limited time that is available to him. It is a sense of inner depletion, impotence, and frustration coupled with the appraisal that his environment offers very little that is inspiring or rewarding.

Perhaps Cumming and Henry have projected into the minds of elderly people the sort of outlook on time and death that they themselves believe to be reasonable and appropriate. This is one of the pitfalls of those who deal with the aged, but most aged people are not theoreticians and simply do not develop the kind of perspective that comes naturally to a theoretician's mind.

Also, we have learned from a number of aged people that they are likely to experience a double-bind regarding time—there is an awareness that future time is scarce but also a heavy sense of oppression at the hands of the clock, too much time that they cannot put to satisfying use. Even a heartfelt lament about the uselessness of future time is not identical with a will-to-die.

Finally, for at least some aged people, the qualitative nature of the future has changed radically. It is no longer the time in which exciting, fresh, novel events are to be expected. The future, in a sense, may be regarded as "used up" before it occurs. The past wends its way forward into the future.

Other points that have emerged from research and clinical experience include:

1. A foreshortened perspective at any age is likely to increase the probability of premature death. The specific pathway of lethality may be through suicide or accident, but particular attention should be given to what might be called psychosomatic or subintentional suicides, in which the individual's physical vulnerabilities are self-exploited to hasten his death.

2. The balance between perspective and engrossment becomes increasingly difficult to maintain with advanced age. An environment that truly shelters the aged person, that truly protects him during his periods of special vulnerability, would make it possible for him to enjoy the spirit-replenishing experience of engrossment more frequently. We become more vulnerable when we are engrossed. We could help our elders if we developed ways of enabling them to drop the burden of their perspectives from time to time without excessive physical or social danger.

3. The perspective of the aged person may become more diffuse or even collapse. Changes in the direction of simplification may be appropriate and

beneficial to some people. But there is the danger that the entire perspective may become dysfunctional and contribute to an unnecessarily steep decline in social integration and behavioral competency. There are things we can do that are likely to have a bolstering effect on the aged person's perspectivistic system. For example, we could enter his past as an active force, a sort of participant-observer. Too often, the aged person's preoccupation with his past chases us away—he is snubbing us by focusing upon a scene in which we had no role. We can develop a sort of semirole in his past and, through this, help him to link his past with the present that all of us share and the future that most of us expect. We are also likely to gain something ourselves through this interpenetration of life perspectives.

4. Both our formal and informal socialization processes emphasize personal growth and expansion during the early years of life. "The System" ill prepares us for living within limits, living with losses, and living with the prospect of death. When the achievement-oriented socialization system gets to work on a person who is growing up in a deprived or ruptured environment, he is alerted to the incongruity between the ideal and the reality. His reaction may take the form of a refusal to accept the socially-sponsored perspective, in the first place, or a rapid aging of the perspective if he does try it out. The person who is growing up in an environment that makes the goals of "The System" appear attractive and feasible is, of course, more likely to develop a life perspective that is centered around individual achievement in the usual sense of the term. Both kinds of people would be better served if our socialization processes—including the classroom—offered a broader, more versatile, and more humane model from which the individual could fashion his own life perspective.

The author gratefully acknowledges the support of the University of Michigan–Wayne State University Institute of Gerontology.

The blacklands of gerontology*

JACQUELYNE JOHNSON JACKSON, Ph.D.**

Previous visits to *The Blacklands of Gerontology* (Jackson, 1967; 1971a) have focused largely upon a presentation and critique of selected literature pertinent to aging and aged blacks, emphasizing especially the paucity *and* inconclusive findings of much of the available data, emergent issues arising therefrom (such as those of relationships between and among race, aging, religion, family and kinship, and health, as well as methodological ones principally concerned with inadequate conceptualizations and collection and interpretation of the data), the usually low socioeconomic statuses of black aged, and critical research and social policy needs. This third visit falls within the same genre, since it provides an additional bibliographic collection and commentary. It also permits a limited assessment of trends in research and factors affecting research on black aged, 1950-1971.

The state of the literature

In general, *The Blacklands of Gerontology* are more fertile than they were two decades ago as there has been a continuing and slowly proliferating

Reproduced from Aging and Human Development 2(3):156-171, 1971.
*This paper was partially supported by the U. S. Public Health Service, Grant #MH1655402, and by the Center for the Study of Aging and Human Development, Duke University Medical Center, Durham, North Carolina, Grant 5 TO1 HD00164 of the National Institute of Child Health and Human Development.
**Assistant professor of medical sociology, Department of Psychiatry, Duke University Medical Center, Durham, North Carolina. Special acknowledgement is made of the bibliographic and other assistance rendered especially by Shirley Bagley (NICHD); Henry Norwood and Peter Hobbes (research assistants); the National Center for Health Statistics, under the directions of Dr. Theodore Woolsey; Daniel I. Rubenstein (Brandeis University); Robert Kastenbaum (Wayne State University); and Viola E. Jackson (my daughter who entertained herself begrudgingly so that I could complete this task).

availability of more heterogeneous literature on black aged. More black subjects are being included in study populations containing white subjects, with a tendency (still conspicuously absent in some cases) of increasing sampling sizes to permit more sophisticated data analyses by race, as well as the very important trend of restricting samples to black subjects alone. This allows isolation of similarities and differences among processes of black aging, clearly recognizing (as many still do not) that blacks are highly variable.

A greater emphasis and concern is being given to minority aged (including blacks) by The Gerontological Society, as exemplified by its sponsorship of roundtable discussions on minorities at recent annual meetings and the special series of articles on elderly minorities in *The Gerontologist,* 11:26-98, 1971. The National Council on Aging has also pursued field work among minority elderly funded largely by the office of Economic Opportunity, and focused on them at its Annual Conference, March, 1971. The Institute of Gerontology at The University of Michigan-Wayne State University shows increased inclusion of minority group students in training programs and recently held a Symposium on "Triple Jeopardy: The plight of Age Minorities in America," April, 1971. The Gerontological Center at the University of Southern California has been making training contributions, sought involvement in various community programs, and developed a Workshop of Ethnicity, Mental Health, and Aging. The significant contributions of the U. S. Senate Special Committee on Aging under the direction of William Oriol include its temporary contract with Dr. Inabel Lindsay to provide a systematic review of available knowledge on black aged.

A small but growing band of black gerontologists and other blacks interested in the aged has emerged.* There has been continuing interest and activities underfoot by the National Urban League to conduct research on and promote concern for the black aged. There is a strong possibility that the Administration on Aging, U. S. Department of Health, Education, and Welfare, will fund, for the first time, a gerontological training program at a black institution (probably at Fisk University where adequate personnel are already available and/or Tennessee State University, both in Nashville) which should contribute significantly

---

*I am often among those asked to identify black gerontologists and/or those behavorial scientists interested in aging. A partial listing would include Dr. Stanley H. Smith (Fisk University); Dr. James E. Blackwell (University of Massachusetts at Boston); Dr. Maurice Jackson (University of Southern California); Dr. Robert Staples (University of California, Irvine); Miss Gloria Walker and Mrs. Marguerite Howie (South Carolina State College); Dr. Wilbur Watson (Rutgers University and the Stephen Smith Geriatric Center, Philadelphia); Dr. Hubert Ross (Atlanta University); Dr. Jesse Gloster (Texas Southern University); Dr. Barbara Solomon (University of Southern California); Dr. James E. Conyers (Indiana State University, Terre Haute); Dr. Ralph H. Hines (Meharry Medical College); Dr. Adelbert H. Jenkins (New York University); Dr. Charles U. Smith (Florida A. and M. University); Dr. Floyd Wylie (Wayne State University); Dr. Robert Hill (National Urban League, Washington, D.C.); Dr. Inabel Lindsay (Washington, D.C.); Mr. Abraham Davis, Jr. (HEW, Washington, D.C.); Dr. Percil Stanford; and Mrs. Mercerdee Thompson (St. Louis).

towards a reduction of the shortage of trained black researchers and service-providers.

A *Research Conference on Minority Group Aged in the South* is planned, to be funded by the National Institute of Child Health and Development, to permit a systematic assessment of the current status of research on the black aged, tentatively scheduled for early October, Nashville, Tennessee. Perhaps the most important development is the formation of the *National Caucus on the Black Aged* in November, 1970, under the leadership of Hobart C. Jackson (Chief Administrator, the Stephen Smith Geriatric Center, Philadelphia) and Robert J. Kastenbaum (Director, Center for the Study of Death, Dying and Lethal Behavior, Wayne State University).

It is significant that those responsible for planning the forthcoming 1971 White House Conference on Aging failed to provide for policy formulations focusing specifically upon the acute problems and needs of minority group aged, especially those who are in "quadruple jeopardy" by being black and female and old and poor. This glaring omission particularly as it relates to critical needs in the areas of housing, income, health and retirement roles and activities, should be corrected. A step in this direction may well be a possible *National Conference on Black Aged,* tentatively scheduled for Washington, D.C., November, 1971. The organization of an effective and permanent "Committee of One Hundred Elderly Black Statesmen," composed largely of those sixty-five or more years of age who have had active professional and civic careers, could do much to spark the needed attention upon the deplorable plight of many black elderly. It would certainly provide a "Black House" of cogent policies for legislative and other remedies.

Despite the fertility of *The Blacklands of Gerontology,* certain critical research, training, and service needs remain extant. These have been identified, particular by Bourg (1971), Havighurst (1971), H. Jackson (1971), J. Jackson (1967; 1970; 1971a; 1971b; 1971c), Jenkins (1971), Kalish (1971), Kastenbaum (1971), and Kent (1971a; 1971b; 1971c), as well as the issue of the implications of recent black militancy on the psychological well-being of aged blacks dividing Elam (1970) and Solomon (1970). These attest to the need for carefully executed, intensive, interdisciplinary studies employing national, random samples of aging and aged blacks. Also needed are an enlarged cadre of gerontologists (especially black) focusing upon black aged, substantial training and research funds for this research, crucial improvements in the services available to black aged, and their satisfactory utilization of such services. Almost all of the behavioral scientists cited recognize the critical and varying impacts of racial discrimination upon aging.

This literature review, with some notable exceptions, is restricted to what has become available within the last several years, as well as certain projections about what is likely to be available within the next year. The search is not exhaustive, and additional information on existing and projected literature and demonstration and service projects would be particularly welcomed. The four areas to be investigated in this review are aging and: (a) health, life expectancy, and race; (b) psychology and race; (c) social patterns, policies, and resources; and (d) additional related information.

Health, life expectancy, and race

The bulk of the literature under consideration relates directly or indirectly to: (1) physical and mental health; (2) factors affecting the delivery and utilization of health-care services; (3) racial differentials in body age, life expectancy, and mortality; and (4) aged sexual behavior.

Physical and mental health. All available data tend to suggest that black males seventy-five or more years of age tend to be in better health than their female or white counterparts. This fact may be attributed to the much earlier deaths of black males who were physiologically, psychologically, and socio-culturally less advantaged. Aging blacks are afflicted by various health disabilities associated with increasing age. However there is still need for a careful study of their physical and mental health in later years.

The National Center for Health Statistics has published some limited but useful data on health patterns of blacks. Included in the most recent National Health Surveys, beginning around 1959, are statistics from medical examinations performed upon a probability sample of noninstitutionalized persons, eighteen to seventy-nine years of age, and later with the Health Interview Surveys. Plans are underfoot to examine the available data systematically. Table 1 provides some selected data on health characteristics of black and white males and females in varying age groupings. These data from the National Health Examination Survey tend to support the expected racial variations in health conditions. They also reveal certain interesting lineal and curvilineal variations by age, sex, and race.

Perhaps one of the most impressive statistics is the finding that a far larger proportion of blacks of both sexes needed dental care than was true of whites—impressive if it points toward the establishment of "Denticare" for the aged. However, the average simplified oral hygiene index is better for black males, seventy-five to seventy-nine years of age than for white males of corresponding ages. Also *fewer* edentulous persons, sixty-five to seventy-four years of age, were found among the blacks than the whites.

Rheumatoid arthritis was more prevalent among females than among the males of both races. With the exception of black males, osteoarthritis tended to increase with age. For the black males, osteoarthritis was curvilineally related to age.

Definite heart disease was more prevalent among blacks than whites and females than males, with the exception of those seventy-five to seventy-nine years of age. Coronary heart disease was more prevalent among whites, while hypertensive heart disease was more typical of blacks. Curvilineal rates by age

Table 1. Selected statistics from the National Health Survey, 1960-1962, by race, sex, and age*

Health characteristic	Black males	Black females	White males	White females
Average simplified oral hygiene index				
Total, 18-79 years	2.4−	2.0−	1.7−	1.3−
55-64 years	2.8−	2.7−	1.9−	1.4−
65-74 years	3.3−	2.5−	2.3−	1.6−
75-79 years	2.7−	2.1−	4.6−	1.5−
Mean no. of decayed, missing, and filled teeth, including edentulous				
persons, Total, 18-79 years	12.9	15.7	20.6	21.9
55-64 years	18.4	25.4	21.2	26.2
65-74 years	23.7	26.9	25.2	27.9
Prevalence rates of edentulous persons				
Total, 18-79 years	7.8	17.7	14.3	20.6
55-64 years	19.5	37.0	29.1	39.1
65-74 years	36.3	45.8	60.7	52.8
Average periodontal index, Total, 18-79 years	1.8−	1.4−	1.3−	0.8−
Percent of dentulous adults needing early dental care, Total, 18-79 years	65.9	57.5	42.9	32.7
55-64 years	78.5	79.2	46.4	31.3
Mean serum cholesterol levels,*				
55-64 years	230	243	234	265
65-74 years	224	266	230	267
Prevalence of rheumatoid arthritis, Rate/100 Adults, Total, 18-79 years	1.5	4.7	1.7	4.6
Prevalence rates (Per 100 adults) for all degrees, Osteoarthritis, Total,				
18-79 years	39.4	34.5	37.8	37.8
55-64 years	66.3	66.4	63.4	75.9
65-74 years	55.6	75.9	77.5	85.7
75-79 years	78.6	78.0	81.1	90.6
Prevalence of definite heart disease				
% Total, 18-79 years	23.8	24.8	11.5	12.5
% 55-64 years	41.6	52.2	22.5	23.7
% 65-74 years	56.9	70.1	31.3	43.5
% 75-79 years	32.3	69.5	39.3	44.8

− = the higher the score the less desirable; + = the lower, the less desirable.
*All data projected for the United States population, 18-79 years of age, with the specific exception of that for mean serum cholesterol levels, which applies only to the sampled whites and the Southern blacks in the Health Examination Survey.
Source: U. S. Public Health Service, National Center for Health Statistics. "Vital and Health Statistics," Data from the National Health Survey, "Series 11,#3, 5, 6, 7, 9, 10, 12, 13, 15, 16, 17, 18, 22, 23, 24, 25, 26, 27, 34, 36, and 37."

Table 1. Selected statistics from the National Health Survey, 1960-1962, by race, sex, and age—cont'd

Health characteristic	Black males	Black females	White males	White females
Prevalence rates (per 100 adults) of definite coronary heart disease,				
Total, 18-79 years	3.2	2.0	3.8	2.1
55-64 years	5.7	5.5	10.3	4.7
65-74 years	3.4	5.1	12.2	8.2
Prevalence rates of definite hypertensive heart disease,				
% Total, 18-79 years	19.1	22.2	6.5	9.8
% 55-64 years	33.1	46.4	11.7	19.5
% 65-74 years	50.2	66.4	16.3	37.5
% 75-79 years	32.3	69.5	24.0	37.1
Percent reactive to the KRP syphilis test				
Total, 18-79 years	22.9	16.3	2.3	2.1
55-64 years	31.0	35.2	3.5	4.1
65-74 years	32.6	13.1	4.0	2.4
Mean systolic blood pressures in mm. hg.				
Total, 18-79 years	136.2	136.3	130.6	129.4
55-64 years	148.3	155.7	139.7	145.8
65-74 years	158.3	175.2	147.1	159.2
75-79 years	156.5	162.8	154.1	156.5
Mean diastolic blood pressures in mm. hg.				
Total, 18-79 years	83.3	83.2	78.3	77.5
55-64 years	89.3	91.9	82.6	84.2
65-74 years	86.9	89.7	80.5	83.3
75-79 years	84.9	82.9	78.9	79.1
Mean blood hematocrit, ml. %				
Total, 18-79 years	45.8+	40.8+	46.5+	42.5+
55-64 years	44.2+	42.1+	46.3+	42.1+
65-74 years	44.1+	41.9+	45.9+	43.3+
Mean glucose levels in mg. %				
Total, 18-79 years	118.5	126.1	115.4	126.5
55-64 years	131.7	141.9	130.2	145.5
65-74 years	150.8	166.2	139.0	159.5
75-79 years	201.1	187.2	151.6	177.5
Distance Vision, 20/20 or better Uncorrected Acuity, Rate/100				
adults, Total, 18-79 years	60.0	52.9	57.3	50.4
55-64 years	23.0	12.9	25.1	17.8
65-74 years	15.3	10.2	8.8	2.4
Near Vision, 14/14 or better Uncorrected Acuity, Rate/100				
adults, Total, 18-79 years	47.8	45.6	47.3	26.7

Continued.

Table 1. Selected statistics from the National Health Survey, 1960-1962, by race, sex, and age—cont'd

Health characteristic	Black males	Black females	White males	White females
Hearing Level (—5dB or less at 1000 cycles/second) Rate/100 population, Total, 18-79 years	62.3	63.2	56.1	60.8
55-64 years	38.8	47.7	44.8	36.1
65-74 years	27.7	32.6	25.1	24.2
75-79 years	30.1	10.2	10.2	8.9
Prevalence of Self-reported Nervous Breakdowns				
% Total, 18-79 years	2.8	10.4	3.2	6.0
% 18-79 years	4.2	24.4	5.6	11.6
% 65-74 years	8.2	23.5	5.2	9.7

characterized coronary and hypertensive heart patterns among the blacks and the latter among white females. Mean serum cholesterol levels were higher for females than for males, whites than for blacks.

The proportion of subjects reactive to the KRP test for syphilis tended to increase with age among all but white females. Mean blood pressure rates were curvilineal with age among blacks and white females. The systolic was lineal and the diastolic, curvilineal among white males. Both black and white males at all age levels had higher mean blood hematocrit levels than was the case for the females, with the latter displaying increases in the later age stages as opposed to decreases among the remaining groups.

Diabetic conditions were more typical among blacks. Mean glucose levels were higher than among the whites for those seventy-five to seventy-nine years of age, with definite lineal increases by age among each group. Black male rates were lower than those of black females until age seventy-five; then the pattern reversed.

In general, a higher proportion of blacks in the late age stages maintained better visual acuity and hearing levels than did whites. The hearing levels of black males, especially those of seventy-five to seventy-nine years of age, tended to be much better than those of their white counterparts. Racial differentiations among the females were not as clear.

Self-reported nervous breakdown data revealed higher proportions among black females than any of the others at all age levels. Special attention should be given to eliciting causal factors contributing to almost 25 percent of black females, fifty-five or more years of age, reporting a nervous breakdown. Some might argue that such self-reported data is unreliable, but it is important to investigate the *meaning* of a situation assigned by the actors involved as well as the so-called objective investigators.

Other data on such variables as chronic conditions, hospitalization, medical visits, and mortality are also available and under systematic investigation. Walker (1970) utilized secondary data in her investigation of relationships between reported chronic ailments and socioeconomic status of the inner-city aged of Nashville, Tennessee. Most of the black and white subjects reported few ailments, but those most often reported revealed certain sex and social class differences. Modal ailments were heart and circulatory disorders among the males, arthritic and other bone disorders among black females, and both skin and arthritic and other bone disorders among white females.

Hypotheses suggested for future investigations are worth noting: (a) the "lower the SES level, the greater the likelihood of a subject feeling ill; (b) there is no significant variation by race for most chronic ailments; (c) where there is such a difference, black females are far more likely to report (or to have) ailments at least partially induced by stress and strain; and therefore (d) both blacks and females are more likely to be affected adversely by the external environment than are white males." (Walker, pp. 50-51.)

The higher rates of perceived nervous breakdowns among black females have already been noted, as well as their greater institutionalized rates in state mental institutions in the late age stages. Mental health in old age may be affected in a number of ways. One of the most important issues now being raised in the literature in this respect is the aforementioned one of the impacts of increased black militancy upon the self-images of older blacks. Moore's (1971) failure to realize what is probably the compatibility of Elam (1970) and Solomon's (1970) positions may be due to a tendency to overgeneralize about blacks. Both positions make sense; they must be applied to the subpopulations rather than the total population. A continuing issue about the mental health of the aged is that of their ability to cope with the addition of age discrimination after having already been subjected to racial discrimination throughout their lives. Careful study is also needed here, for data are highly inconclusive (cf. Jackson, 1967 and Moore, 1971).

Factors affecting the delivery and utilization of health-care services. The work of Fabrega, et al. (1969) and Gordon and Rehr (1969) point to some of the problems affecting adequate delivery and utilization of such services. What is most important are their stresses upon the attitudes of care-givers in making distinctions and certain apparent ethnic differences in reaching out for assistance when in need. Probably the most important implication is that black aged, in particular, need increasing awareness of the medical system so as to adapt better to it and make it adapt better to them.

Racial differences in body age, life expectancy, and mortality. The most exciting for me is Morgan's (1968) finding that differential physical aging among black and white males tends to justify assumptions that black males are indeed old earlier than white males:

> Negro males of 30 calendar years on have an older body age than their white counterparts. The biggest jump in body age is between 21 and 30, after which Negroes hold a 5-yr. body-age differential until 60 (then increasing further) (p. 598).

Such a finding provides further support for differential minimum age-eligibility requirements for recipients of *Old-Age Assistance, Survivors, Disability, and Health Insurance* (OASDHI) so as to reflect racial differentials in life expectancies (Jackson, 1970; 1971c) and, now, body ages.

Additional support is garnered in Demeny and Gingrich's (1967) careful critique of American black-white mortality differentials:

> Unless it is assumed that age patterns of death for United States Negroes were extremely deviant from those found in populations with reliable census and vital statistics, one must conclude that the official figures grossly underestimate early childhood mortality for Negroes, at least for the period, 1910-1940. It follows that, during those decades, *Negro-white mortality differentials in terms of expectation of life at birth were also substantially higher than is suggested by the official estimates* (p. 820, *italics added*).

Finally, Hill (1971) has pointed out that recently the life expectancy for black males has *decreased*. That may be affected by the increases noted in infant mortality among blacks in certain metropolitan areas over the past decade.

Aged sexual behavior. In their mortality and survival comparisons of black eunuchs and intact persons in a mentally retarded population in Kansas, Hamilton and Mestler (1969) suggested that the eunuchs tended to survive longer, but the significant difference found among the comparable whites did not appear among the blacks:

> The difference between eunuchs and intact men with regard to duration of life was significantly more in whites than in non-whites (13.5 vs. 3 years). The detrimental effects of testicular function upon viability, and the benefit from orchiectomy, may prove to be more in white than in non-white males (p. 410).

As in other studies, the small sampling size of the blacks tended to prohibit more elaborate data analyses.

Pfeiffer, Verwoerdt, and Wang (1968; 1969) included blacks in their analyses of aged sexual behavior, most often without racial separation of the data. They held that the "Negro and white Ss did not differ significantly from one another in respect to age-related patterns of sexual interest and activity" (p. 197). If so, their findings are supportive of other accumulating data which refute the notion of "black sexual bestiality." They did indicate the need to study subjects under sixty years of age, and especially women, so as to amass more information on sexual behavior and aging. It would be very interesting to determine whether earlier decreases in sexual behavior tended to occur among black females then white females when they are subjected to more years without a spouse.

Psychology and race

Most psychological literature on the aged has avoided the utilization of black subjects. Where they have been utilized, the problems under investigation have been perceived as unaffected by race. Recent literature has shifted some attention to the dynamics of race and age, with the most significant being that of Kastenbaum (1971), Jenkins (1971), and Brunswick (1969-1970).

Kastenbaum's (1971) investigation of differential attitudes toward future optimism and subjective life expectancies among young black and old whites is most intriguing. Noting the foreshortened time perspective typical of deprived, depressed, aged, or dying subjects, he has applied this model to *hard-core unemployed* black males recruited for participation in a job opportunity program (Teahan and Kastenbaum, 1970). Comparisons of those who remained in and who left the program at one and six month intervals led him to the formulation of an hypothesis under further investigation: "there is at least a partial functional equivalence between the phenomenologic world of young-and-black and the old-and-white." Incidentally, this study also appears promising in the accumulation of more data attesting to the earlier *oldness* occurring among black, than among white males.

Jenkins (1971) has employed an Eriksonian model in providing therapeutic treatment to a young black male experiencing life-adjustment difficulties, and has suggested that racial factors prohibiting adequate achievement of ego integrity in the earlier years are dysfunctionally related to mature adaptation to old age. Thus, he emphasizes the necessity to reform society so as to promote healthier aging among blacks.

Brunswick's (1969-70) analysis of black and white intergenerational differences in outlook on life, interracial tolerance and hostility, and attitudes toward advocacy of violence note especially differential attitudes among younger and older subjects. She has stressed her belief that "education is at least as important a divider, or determiner of generations, as age" (p. 369), and her article is fraught with implications for further investigations of possible generation gaps by age and other variables among blacks and whites. I suspect that self-concept may well be an important divider among blacks.

Byrne's, et al. (1969) findings about the relative universality of responding positively to strangers expressing attitudes similar to one's own and negatively to those bearing dissimilar attitudes portends significant implications for relationships in direct services to the elderly especially, and could, perhaps, be tied in with the Thune (1969) studies of racial attitudes among white and black subjects in a Nashville Senior Citizens Center.

Social patterns, policies, and resources

The bulk of the recent literature falls within the areas of social patterns, policies, and resources. Demographic aspects are also of interest, given the projected data from the U. S. Bureau of the Census (and a possibility that a

Table 2. Percentage of persons 65 or more years of age within the total black population, by sex and state, 1970

State	Males	Females	State	Males	Females
West Virginia	14.2	13.7	Michigan	5.4	5.9
Arkansas	11.8	12.5	Maryland	5.3	6.0
Oklahoma	9.6	10.8	Illinois	5.2	5.9
Mississippi	9.3	10.1	Oregon	5.2	5.2
Kentucky	9.3	11.1	Wyoming	4.9	6.5
Alabama	8.6	10.3	District of Columbia	4.8	6.2
Tennessee	8.5	9.6	Massachusetts	4.7	6.0
Kansas	7.9	9.6	New Jersey	4.7	5.8
Missouri	7.8	8.7	Rhode Island	4.7	6.7
Louisiana	7.5	8.8	New Mexico	4.7	4.9
Texas	7.5	8.5	New York	4.5	5.8
Pennsylvania	7.1	7.9	California	4.3	5.5
Virginia	6.7	8.2	Idaho	4.2	3.9
Iowa	6.7	7.6	Montana	4.1	5.5
Arizona	6.6	6.6	Maine	4.0	5.9
Ohio	6.4	7.0	Colorado	3.8	5.9
North Carolina	6.3	7.8	Washington	3.7	4.4
Georgia	6.2	8.5	Utah	3.6	6.9
Florida	6.0	6.9	Connecticut	3.5	4.5
Indiana	6.0	6.8	Wisconsin	3.2	3.4
South Carolina	5.7	7.7	South Dakota	3.1	4.0
Delaware	5.7	6.5	Nevada	3.0	3.2
Nebraska	5.6	6.5	New Hampshire	2.5	3.2
Vermont	5.6	6.9	Alaska	1.1	1.4
Minnesota	5.4	6.3	North Dakota	0.8	1.0
			Hawaii	0.8	1.2

Source of raw data: U. S. Bureau of the Census. Advance Report, United States, General Population Characteristics, PC(V2)-1, U. S. Department of Commerce, Washington, D.C., February, 1971.

special report on black aged in the fifty largest cities may be forthcoming from that agency).

In 1970, the reported 1,565,897 blacks, sixty-five or more years of age, represented an increase of about one-third percent over those reported in 1960. As expected, most (56.7%) were females, and most (60.8%) resided in the South. North Dakota had the fewest (twelve males and ten females), while New York had the largest number of females (67,509), and Texas, the largest number of males (50,965). Table 2 contains data on the proportion of blacks sixty-five or more years of age within each state. As shown, West Virginia had both the largest proportion of males and females, while Hawaii and North Dakota had the least.

Hill (1971) has detailed available recent demographic characteristics of the black aged, noting especially their patterns of residence, marital statuses and household compositions, income, education, employment, and health. Of special significance is the fact that he plans to provide a succinct demographic analysis when sufficient data are available. Herman Brotman (Administration on Aging) is also in the process of continuing his highly competent compilation of statistical data on the aged, including black aged, and will be providing information particularly about changes within the last decade. Finally, Inabel Lindsay (Member, Task Force on Problems of the Aging, appointed by President Richard M. Nixon, 10 October 1969) was in the process of summarizing available information on black aged in her role as a temporary consultant to the U. S. Senate Special Committee on Aging (a role which occurred as one of the responses to the *National Caucus on the Black Aged*). All of these compilations will attest to the continued generally low socioeconomic statuses of black aged, and, perhaps, to a slightly rising rate of institutionalization among them.

Utilization of Census and the National Center for Health Statistics data clearly point to the need, as Kent has implied (1971a), for substantially enlarged sample sizes involving blacks, so as to permit far more sophisticated data analyses. Also, given the nature of the times and the need to "check out" the rapidity of change, national data collected at at least five-year intervals (instead of decennially) and reported separately (i.e., not as "nonwhite") for blacks would be of great value. The racial separation apparent in the last few years is a welcome step in the right direction.

Familial, kinship, and retirement roles. Major research developments include the likelihood of publication of data from the Philadelphia Aged Services Project under the direction of Donald P. Kent, and from J. Jackson's "Roles and resources of older, urban blacks" (should I cease writing reviews!) within the next year. Such publications will tend to document specific kinship patterns, as well as other data, among urban blacks in Philadelphia, Pennsylvania, and Durham, North Carolina, respectively. As far as I know no similar studies involving rural aged blacks are underway (in fact, I have not yet located a recent research study on them). These sets of expected publications will probably emphasize strengths and weaknesses of specific subgroups of aged blacks, and the Philadelphia series will provide racial comparisons, and emphasize the feasibility of a network of "caretakers" often found and trained among deprived populations. I wish to again stress my belief that the Philadelphia study can provide an excellent model of "how-to-do-research," for its concerns have not been merely with collecting data, but with providing assistance to the subjects!

My data on kinship patterns and processes among predominantly low-income urban black aged reveal primarily their effective kinship networks or substitutes. They also provide specific information on relationships with parents, children, siblings, grandchildren, cousins, and best friends. The preliminary report on grandparent-grandchild interaction (Jackson, 1971c) shows that the grandparental subjects preferred grandchildren living near them (but not with them) and younger (rather than older) grandchildren. Relationships among their affectional closeness, value consensus, and identification with their grandchildren were unclear, but preferences did appear to be related to particular grandchild types. The data also suggested the implausibility of a general postulation of a "generation gap," because age proved to be a highly insufficient variable, particularly among the males. The findings also debunked the usual myths about disintegrating black families, while sustaining the picture of the important roles many of them actually serve as "Individual Departments of Welfare" when the society fails to provide adequate education, employment, income, and housing for themselves, their children, and their children's children.

"Sex and social class variations in black older parent-adult child relationships" (Jackson, 1971b) did reveal certain significant differences found among a pilot sample of largely middle-class aged blacks in Durham. While most of the parental subjects received some instrumental assistance from children, middle-class parents were more likely than lower-class parents to receive this assistance, and, as expected, daughters tended to be more likely than sons to provide it. The study also suggests the need for greater analysis of parental-child sex preferences in black families.

A most impressive research study in process, particularly by virtue of its utilization of a national sample (3,340 whites and 487 blacks) is that undertaken by Rubenstein (1971). His comparisons of the social participation—largely familial and kinship, among aged whites and blacks has led him to conclude that there are no racial differences in the proportion of those living alone and isolated and in their emotional state of well-being or morale. He does expect to report finally that the blacks fare more poorly as measured by education, occupation, income, and employment, which is, of course, in agreement with existing findings. Lambing's (1969) study of retired blacks in an urban setting in Florida contributes, as well, to a growing body of highly localized data on aged blacks.

Fillenbaum's (1971) report of relationships between job and retirement attitudes found among nonacademic employees in a North Carolina university and medical center indicated that those relationships were quite minimal. She concluded that "only where work holds the central organizing position in a person's life (which here it does not) should job attitudes influence retirement attitudes" (p. 247). What is of greater significance for present purposes is the finding that the white and black subjects could not be racially distinguished by their attitudes toward retirement. However, she did find a racially significant difference in that the negative association between achievement (i.e., "possible acquisition of further knowledge and skills") and retirement typical of the whites was not typical of the blacks. I could not determine whether this was a spurious finding since she provided no *specific* occupational data on the subjects by race. However, almost all, if not all, of the lower echelon "housekeeping" personnel in the populations under study were black, and almost none of the remaining nonacademic employees were in the upper echelon slots at the time that the data were collected. In other words, further investigation of the finding is warranted.

Housing and social resources. A preliminary report from an analysis of impacts of housing relocation among older blacks (Jackson, 1970) revealed many similarities among applicants to an age-segregated public housing complex, as measured by the Carp Housing Schedule (Carp, 1965). The most significant finding is that of the differences separating the successful and nonsuccessful applicants. Briefly, those who were male, younger, and married were more successful, portending grave implications for black aged, for, in some sense, those who were the least deprived were those most likely to gain acceptance by the white admission agents. It would be unfortunate if the usual pattern of rejecting those blacks most in need of educational, employment, and other opportunities comes to characterize the aged as well.

Bourg (1971) has issued a preliminary report on his ongoing investigation of "Life styles and mobility patterns of older persons in Nashville-Davidson County" (Tennessee). This study is primarily concerned with a description of various settings surrounding the elderly and with developmental processes involved in their psychological and sociocultural aging. Findings from his sample of 297 black aged (no other group is under investigation) emphasize their conspicuous diversity "in the functions provided by their social relationships" and their mobility differences. The second phase utilizes a panel of subjects to obtain more detailed information on "the relationship between mobility patterns with small boundaries and dependence on the immediate environment." His study is of special value in that the restriction to blacks only helped to focus upon their differences. He calls attention to the need to explore "the differences amid the similarities" and "the similar components which emerge among the differences."

Lopata's (1970) study of "Social relations of widows in black and white urban communities" could well benefit from utilizing at least a twofold comparative model: (a) racial comparisons with whites, as she has done; and (b) comparisons holding race constant. Her characterization of the black widows tends to fall within the traditional pathological mold, and one cannot determine readily if the widows themselves were fairly interpreted or if the interpreter unduly influenced her data. Her conceptualization of black widows as being untrained in "skills which facilitate the conversion of strangers into friends" and "often unable to enter any social relation with a great deal of intimacy" (pp. 29-30) represented her value judgement and, perhaps, attests anew to the critical importance of black people performing their own research in such cases. We are given no indication of the variety of black widows located in the Chicago Metropolitan Area.

H. Jackson (1971) has aptly summarized priorities requiring attention to promote the welfare of the aged. The greatest need is for an adequate income, with a minimal floor of $6,000 for an individual and $9,000 per married couple for those sixty-five or more years of age. When necessary, annual adjustments should be made to maintain the equivalent of this income. Other needs given high priority included employment, health, and a nationwide network of community services. In his role as a private citizen and as National Chairman, the National Caucus on the Black Aged, he is committed to strive to achieve these goals.

Related literature

In addition to suggested references covering the topics discussed above, the bibliography contains a section on "Additional related literature" pertinent to those areas. They are primarily concerned with the "generation gap," political involvement of the aged, and the provision of social services, such as in health and transportation.

Summary

This third review of social gerontological literature on black aged has focused largely upon recent developments in available data on health and longevity (including body age), psychology and race, and social patterns, policies and resources, as well as related organizational developments. An increasing number of investigators of and investigations on black aged have appeared within the last few years, but none have yet embarked upon a clearly mandated highly sophisticated, interdisciplinary study involving a *large,* random sample of aging and aged blacks throughout the nation. Also, few of these investigators have been black, but the possibility of the development of a social gerontological training program in research at Fisk University may reduce this problem somewhat, as has, indeed, the significant contributions already made by such institutions as Duke University, The University of Michigan, Wayne State University, and the University of Southern California.

There has been far less interest recently in cataloguing the objective social conditions, and far more interest in studying the processes of aging and the specific environmental conditions of black aged. Greater attention has been given to investigations of the influence of race upon aging (e.g., Kastenbaum, 1971; Jenkins, 1971) and upon differences among black aged (e.g., Bourg, 1971; Jackson, 1970; 1971b). More progress has also been made in identifying commonalities among black and white aging and aged persons (e.g., in Kent's Philadelphia Aged Services Project; Fillenbaum, 1971; Pfeiffer, et al., 1969). Two of the most critical research needs are mental illness among the black aged, and trends in the use or non-use of nursing homes by the black aged.

The formation of the National Caucus on the Black Aged in November, 1970, was very significant. It may well serve as a viable catalyst in producing desired research, training, and services for black and other aged Americans.

While it is no longer true that almost nothing is known about black aged, it is still true that we've got a long way to go! It would be helpful if some of the research, training, and service needs already identified here and elsewhere were executed with greater speed. Finally, it would be extremely helpful if Nathan Shock were to extend his bibliographic captions to include a section on "Minority Group Aged."

SELECTED BIBLIOGRAPHY

I. Health, life expectancy and race

Conley, Ronald W.: "Labor force loss due to disability." Public Health Reports, 84:291-298, 1969.

Demeny, Paul, and Paul Gingrich: "A reconsideration of Negro-white mortality differentials in the United States." Demography, 4:820-837, 1967.

Elam, Lloyd C.: "Critical factors for mental health in aging black populations." Paper delivered at the Workshop of Ethnicity, Mental Health, and Aging, Los Angeles, 1970.

Fabrega, Horacio, Jr., Richard J. Moore, and John R. Strawn: "Low income medical problem patients: some medical and behavioral features." Journal of Health and Social Behavior, 10:334-343, 1969.

Gordon, Barbara, and Helen Rehr: "Selectivity biases in delivery of hospital social services." Social Service Review, 43:35-41, 1969.

Hamilton, James B., and Gordon E. Mestler: "Mortality and survival: comparison of eunuchs with intact men and women in a mentally retarded population." Journal of Gerontology, 24:395-411, 1969.

Metropolitan Life Insurance Company: "Trends in mortality of nonwhites." Statistical Bulletin, 51:5-8, 1970.

Morgan, Robert F.: "The adult growth examination: preliminary comparisons of physical aging in adults by sex and race." Perceptual and motor skills, 27:595-599, 1968.

Pfeiffer, Eric, Adriann Verwoerdt, and Hsioh-Shan Wang: "The natural history of sexual behavior in a biologically advantaged group of aged individuals." Journal of Gerontology, 24:193-198, 1969.

Pfeiffer, Eric, Adriann Verwoerdt, and Hsioh-Shan Wang: "Sexual behavior in aged men and women." Archives of General Psychiatry, 19:753-758, 1968.

Solomon, Barbara: "Ethnicity, mental health and the older black aged." Gerontological Center, University of Southern California, Los Angeles, 1970.

U. S. Department of Health, Education, and Welfare, Public Health Service, National Center for Health Statistics: "Vital and health statistics, Data from the National Health Survey." U. S. Government Printing Office, Washington, D.C.

–: "Binocular visual acuity of adults, United States, 1960-1962," Series 11, Number 3, 1964.

–: "Binocular visual acuity of adults by region and selected demographic characteristics, United States, 1960-1962," Series 11, Number 25, 1967.

–: "Blood glucose levels in adults, United States, 1960-1962," Series 11, Number 18, 1966.

–: "Blood pressure as it relates to physique, blood glucose, and serum cholesterol, United States, 1960-1962," Series 11, Number 34, 1969.

–: "Blood pressure of adults by race and area, United States, 1960-1962," Series 11, Number 5, 1964.

–: "Chronic conditions and limitations of activity and mobility, United States, July, 1965-June, 1967," Series 10, Number 61, 1971.

–: "Coronary heart disease in adults, United States, 1960-1962," Series 11, Number 10, 1965.

–: "Decayed, missing, and filled teeth in adults, United States, 1960-1962," Series 11, Number 23, 1967.

–: "Differentials in health characteristics by color, United States, July, 1965-June, 1967," Series 10, Number 56, 1969.

–: "Family use of health services, United States, July, 1963-June, 1964," Series 10, Number 55, 1969.

–: "Findings on the serologic test for syphilis in adults, United States, 1960-1962," Series 11, Number 9, 1965.

–: "Hearing levels of adults by race, region, and area of residence, United States, 1960-1962," Series 11, Number 26, 1967.

–: "Heart disease in adults, United States, 1960-1962," Series 11, Number 6, 1964.

–: "Hypertension and hypertensive heart disease in adults, United States, 1960-1962," Series 11, Number 13, 1966.

–: "Mean blood hematocrit of adults, United States, 1960-1962," Series 11, Number 24, 1967.

–: "Need for dental care among adults, United States, 1960-1962," Series 11, Number 36, 1970.

–: "Oral hygiene in adults, United States, 1960-1962," Series 11, Number 16, 1966.

–: "Periodontal disease in adults, United States, 1960-1962," Series 11, Number 12, 1965.

–: "Persons hospitalized by number of hospital episodes and days in a year, United States, July, 1965-June, 1966," Series 10, Number 50, 1969.

–: "Persons injured and disability days due to injury, United States, July, 1965-June, 1967," Series 10, Number 58, 1970.

–: "Prevalence of osteoarthritis in adults by age, sex, race, and geographic area, United States, 1960-1962," Series 11, Number 15, 1966.

–: "Prevalence of selected impairments, United States, July, 1963-June, 1965," Series 10, Number 48, 1968.

–: "Rheumatoid arthritis in adults, United States, 1960-1962," Series 11, Number 17, 1966.

–: "Selected dental findings in adults by age, race, and sex, United States, 1960-1962," Series 11, Number 7, 1965.

–: "Serum Cholesterol levels of adults, United States, 1960-1962," Series 11, Number 22, 1967.

–: "Selected symptoms of psychological distress, United States," Series 11, Number 37, 1970.

–: "Total loss of teeth in adults, United States, 1960-1962," Series 11, Number 27, 1967.

–: "Volume of physician visits, United States, July, 1966-June, 1967," Series 10, Number 49, 1968.

Walker, Gloria V.: "The relationship between socioeconomic status and chronic ailments of the aged in Nashville, Tennessee." Unpublished master's thesis, Fisk University, Nashville, Tennessee, 1970.

II. Psychology and race

Brunswick, Ann F.: "What generation gap? A comparison of some generation differences among blacks and whites." Social Problems, 17:358-370, 1969-1970.

Byrne, Donn, William Griffitt, William Hudgins, and Keith Reeves: "Attitude similarity-dissimilarity and attraction: generality beyond the college sophomore." The Journal of Social Psychology, 79:155-161, 1969.

Jenkins, Adelbert H.: "Growth crisis in a young black man: its relationship to family and aging." Paper presented at the annual meeting of the Eastern Psychological Association, New York City, 1971.

Kalish, Richard A.: "A gerontological look at ethnicity, human capacities, and individual adjustment." The Gerontologist, 11:78-87, 1971.

Kastenbaum, Robert J.: "Time without a future: on the functional equivalence between young-and-black and aged-and-white." Paper presented at the annual meeting of the Eastern Psychological Association, New York City, 1971.

Teahan, John, and Robert Kastenbaum: "Subjective Life Expectancy and Future Time Perspective as Predictors of Job Success in the 'Hard-Core Unemployed.' " Omega, 1, No. 3, 189-200, 1970.

Thune, Jeanne M.: "Group portrait in black and white." Senior Citizens, Inc., Nashville, Tennessee, 1969.

III. Social patterns, policies, and resources

Bourg, Carroll: "The changing environment of older persons." Paper presented at the 35th annual meeting of the Association of Social and Behavioral Scientists, Montgomery, Alabama, 1971.

Cohen, Elias S.: "Welfare policies for the aged poor: a contradiction." Paper delivered at the Symposium on Triple Jeopardy: The Plight of Aged Minorities in America. The Institute of Gerontology, The University of Michigan-Wayne State University, Detroit, April, 1971.

Fillenbaum, Gerda G.: "On the relation between attitude to work and attitude to retirement." Journal of Gerontology, 26:244-248, 1971.

Havighurst, Robert J.: "Report of a Conference on Flexible Carreers." The Gerontologist, 11:21-25, 1971.

Hays, David S., and Morris Wisotsky: "The aged offender: a review of the literature and two current studies from the New York State Division of Parole." Journal of the American Geriatric Society, 17:1064-1073, 1969.

Hill, Robert: "A profile of the black aged." Paper delivered at the Symposium on Triple Jeopardy: The Plight of Aged Minorities in America. The Institute of Gerontology, The University of Michigan-Wayne State University, Detroit, April, 1971.

Jackson, Hobart C.: "National goals and priorities in the social welfare of the aging." The Gerontologist, 11:88-94, 1971.

Jackson, Jacquelyne J.: "Social gerontology and the Negro: a review." The Gerontologist, 7:168-178, 1967.

Jackson, Jacquelyne J.: "Social impacts of housing relocation upon urban, low-income, black aged." Paper delivered at the annual meeting of the Gerontological Society, Toronto, Canada, 1970.

Jackson, Jacquelyne J.: "Negro aged: toward needed research in social gerontology." The Gerontologist, 11:52-57, 1971a.

Jackson, Jacquelyne J.: "Sex and social class variations in black older parent-adult child relationships." Aging and Human Development, in press, 1971b.

Jackson, Jacquelyne J.: "Aged blacks: a potpourri in the direction of the reduction of inequities." Phylon, in press, 1971c.

Jackson, Jacquelyne J.: "Compensatory care for aged minorities." Paper delivered at the Symposium on Triple Jeopardy: The Plight of Aged Minorities in America. The Institute of Gerontology, The University of Michigan-Wayne State University, April, 1971d.

Kent, Donald P.: "The delivery of welfare services: reordering the system." Paper delivered at the Symposium on Triple Jeopardy: The Plight of Aged Minorities in America. The Institute of Gerontology, The University of Michigan-Wayne State University, April, 1971b.

Kent, Donald P.: "The elderly in minority groups: variant patterns of aging." The Gerontologist, 11:26-29, 1971a.

Kent, Donald P.: "The Negro aged." The Gerontologist, 11:48-51, 1971c.

Lambing, Mary L.: "A study of retired older Negroes in an urban setting." Unpublished Ph. D. dissertation, University of Florida, Gainesville, 1969.

Lopata, Helena Z.: "Social and family relations of black and white widows in urban communities." Administration on Aging Publication #25, U. S. Department of Health, Education, and Welfare, 1970.

Moore, Joan W.: "Situational factors affecting minority aging." The Gerontologist, **11**:88-93, 1971.

Rubenstein, Daniel I.: "An examination of social participation found among a national sample of black and white elderly." Aging and Human Development, **2**, 1971.

The Gerontologist, **11**:26-98, 1971.

IV. Additional related references

(African aged)

Arth, Malcolm J.: "An interdisciplinary view of the aged in Ibo culture." Journal of Geriatric Psychiatry, **2**:33-39, 1968.

Arth, Malcolm J.: "Ideals and behavior: a comment on Ibo respect patterns." The Gerontologist, **8**:242-244, 1968.

Shelton, Austin J.: "Igbo child-raising, eldership and dependence: further notes for gerontologists and others." The Gerontologist, **8**:236-241, 1968.

(Other references)

Adams, Bert N.: "Isolation, function, and beyond: American kinship in the 1960's." Journal of Marriage and the Family, **32**:575-597, 1970.

Brody, Stanley J., Harvey Finkle, and Carl Hirsch: "Benefit Alert, a public advocacy program for the aged." Paper presented at the 8th International Congress of Gerontology, Washington, D.C., 1969.

Cantor, Marjorie H.: "Elderly ridership and reduced transit fares: the New York City experience." Administration on Aging Publication, #23, U. S. Department of Health, Education, and Welfare.*

Cantor, Marjorie, Karen Rosenthal, and Mary Mayer: "The elderly in the rental market of New York City." Administration on Aging Publication, #26, U. S. Department of Health, Education, and Welfare.*

Carey, Jean Wallace: "Senior advisory service for public housing tenants." Paper delivered at the annual meeting of the Gerontological Society, Toronto, Canada, 1970.

Carp, Frances M.: A future for the aged, Victoria Plaza. The University of Texas Press, Austin, 1966.

Carp, Frances M.: "Public transit and retired people." Administration on Aging Publication, #32, U. S. Department of Health, Education, and Welfare.*

Hoffman, Adeline (ed.): The daily needs and interests of older people. Charles C Thomas, Publisher, Springfield, Illinois, 1970.

McGuire, Marie C.: "The status of housing for the elderly." The Gerontologist, **9**:10-14, 1969.

Shapiro, Sam, Eve Weinblatt, Charles W. Frank, and Robert V. Sager: "Social factors in the prognosis of men following first myocardial infarction." Milbank Memorial Fund Quarterly, **47**:56-63, 1969.

Suchman, Edward A., and A. Allen Rothman: "The utilization of dental services." Milbank Memorial Fund Quarterly, **47**:56-63, 1969.

Trela, James E.: "Age graded secondary association memberships and political involvement in old age." Paper presented at the annual meeting of the Gerontological Society, Toronto, Canada, 1970.

Troll, Lillian E.: "Issues in the Study of Generations." Aging and Human Development, **1**:199-218, 1970.

U. S. Bureau of the Census. "Advance report. General Population Characteristics." PC(V2)-1, U. S. Department of Commerce, Washington, D.C., February, 1971.

---

*It would be helpful if the Administration on Aging Publications were dated.

U. S. Senate. Developments in Aging, 1970, A Report of the Special Committee on Aging, Report No. 92-46, U. S. Government Printing Office, Washington, D.C., 1971.

(References not examined)

Dominick, Joan: "Mental patients in nursing homes: four ethnic influences." Journal of American Geriatric Society, **17**:63+, 1969.

Gregory, R. J.: "A survey of residents in five nursing and rest homes in Cumberland County, North Carolina." Journal of the American Geriatric Society, **18**:501-506, 1970.

10 Eating and aging

LILLIAN E. TROLL, Ph.D.*

In part, this paper is concerned with a dilemma underlying nutritional policy for the aged. The following paragraphs contain one set of statements that point in one direction matched with another set of statements that point in an opposite direction. Consider the first set of propositions:

(a) Eating is one of the most basic ways of living.

(b) The fact of their survival attests to the essential adequacy of the eating practices of old people. And more and more people are living into old age; at present, one out of ten people in the United States are over sixty-five.[1]

(c) Life in old age is much more a continuation of past ways of living than of marked change. The best prediction of what a person will be like when he gets old is that he will be like what he is now, and what he has been up to now, only more so. People seem to get more like themselves as they get older and less like other people. Variance of any characteristic increases, so that there is no such thing as an aged type of person.[2]

All of this suggests that it would be a mistake to adopt any fixed set of rules about diet and eating practices for older people and expect them to be good for *all* old people. In fact, other things being equal—if they ever are—the best eating practices for most older people are probably what they are already practicing. At any rate, it would not be wise for a professional nutritionist to institute any changes in an older person's eating practices before making sure that, first, there is something very wrong with those practices and, second, that the proposed changes are indeed an improvement. (Of course, this rule would apply to all the helping professions, not only those which are involved with nutrition.)

Reproduced from Journal of the American Dietetic Association 59:456-459, November, 1971.
*Wayne State University, Detroit, Michigan.

The other side of the coin

Now consider this other set of statements:

(a) Good food is essential to good health.

(b) The aging body becomes increasingly sensitive and less tolerant; food habits that could once have just produced minor discomforts, or no trouble at all, can cause serious illness in old age. Or, food that once caused pleasure can lead to discomfort.[3]

(c) Aging is usually accompanied by significant activity changes. In fact, one thing we can say for sure about ability and performance changes in the process of aging is that they are all in the direction of slowing down.[4] As we age, we become more sluggish and sedentary, and the food habits we acquired when we were younger, in a time of more abundant exercise and bodily movement, are no longer appropriate to our way of life.

(d) If food has been used as a comforter, there are more and more losses for which comfort is needed, and more and more desire for food the nourishment from which could well be dispensed with. The cost of survival is the outliving of many of the things that made life worth living. Those who live the longest necessarily experience the loss of most of the people they love, of most of their social involvements, and of most of the landmarks of existence that tell them who they are and where they have come from.

(e) Food costs money. Few old people in this country today raise their own food; they must buy it. Yet almost one-fourth of older Americans (over sixty-five) are poor and nearly all feel a squeeze on their fixed incomes.[5] Howell and Loeb state[3]: "A significant proportion of adults over the age of 65 in the United States do not have incomes adequate to purchase . . . a diet which provides for health and well-being" (p. 7). While not all old people are poor (and some are very rich indeed), for those who are poor, the buying of food either on the basis of past habits or on the basis of present optimal nutrition may be impossible. Something must be dropped. When a meat and potatoes and fruit family drops the meat and the fruit and keeps the potatoes because they are cheaper, there has been tremendous qualitative deterioration in their diet as a whole. A good diet is a *gestalt,* a whole combination of foods. If some foods are dropped for reasons of economy, the good effect is gone.

(f) Economy is not the only reason for dropping part of a diet. Lack of energy for shopping and for preparing certain foods is another important contributor to subtle but consequential changes in a diet *gestalt.* Whether this lessened energy comes from loss of vigor, from depression, or even in a circular way from loss of previous good eating habits, it leads to distortion of the nutritional pattern.

There is thus a primary contradiction between what in all probability is a proven good way of eating—proven by the fact of survival—and the physical and social changes that might make some of the past good ways no longer so good.

Two broad issues involved in evaluating the eating of the aging are the social nature of eating on one hand and the isolating consequences of aging on the other.

The process of aging

Let us consider the general process of aging. Just as there is wide variation among individuals in time and speed of development, both toward early maturity and on into the later phases of the life cycle, so there is wide variation in time and speed of development and aging within any individual among bodily systems and social and psychologic processes. Vision, for example, starts aging at birth. But most biologic processes, such as strength, quick thinking, sexual power, or general vigor, increase from birth through childhood and adolescence to a high point in the twenties, followed by an apparent plateau through the years of maturity and middle age to a relatively slow decline thereafter. Other abilities, e.g., athletic, start to decline almost from the time of greatest power, in the middle twenties, and this decline usually proceeds rapidly. Still other abilities show no noticeable decrease until the very end of life; they may even exhibit a steady continuous increase. This is the case for the accumulation of information and vocabulary.[6,7]

Over the years, intelligence tests of populations of all ages have shown a steady increase in intelligence (I.Q.) to some time in the teens or the twenties with a steady decrease thereafter.[4,7] This has been widely interpreted as indicating that people lose their intellectual capacity from about the age of twenty—a most depressing thought. There are several signs of hope, however. First, the correlation of intelligence, as measured by these intelligence tests, with amount of education is very high. This means that if one has more education, his intelligence tends to be higher and to stay higher longer. And the educational level of the American population has been increasing steadily over the last century.

Second, the age at which the decline in intelligence is said to begin has been rising progressively over the years of research. A generation ago, the peak of intelligence was stated as twelve, then it rose to seventeen, then to about twenty-three, then to about thirty, then fifty, and a recent report shows no significant drop before seventy. [8]

It is important to note, though, that the one function that clearly decreases throughout maturity and old age is speed, and anything involving speed—and, of course, almost everything does involve speed—will show decline early. Slowing down starts in the twenties or at least the thirties. On the other hand, capacities that involve accumulation and storage of experience, e.g., vocabulary and information, show increases throughout the life span until just before death. Thus, it now looks as if early findings about intellectual decreases (which, incidentally had been based on cross-sectional rather than the more appropriate longitudinal research) were more likely measuring secular trends in education of the population rather than decline in intelligence. If necessary, old people can learn new ways, particularly if given time.

It is useful to think of three kinds of aging: physical aging, social aging, and psychologic aging. They may not necessarily be in step. For example, it is possible to be physically aged in the forties, but at the same time, socially middle aged and psychologically young. A college professor who is keen of mind, at the height of social involvement, but with little physical activity would fit this description. It is equally possible to be physically middle aged in the seventies, socially young, and psychologically old. A vigorous golfer with many friends and few social responsibilities whose thinking has become rigid and slow would fit this combination. At another extreme, it is possible to be physically alive but socially and psychologically dead. This is true of old and not-so-old patients in mental hospitals, chronic hospitals, or nursing homes. It is also true of many older people living in their children's homes and having no social role or function there.

From earliest life, eating is a social activity, embedded in a complex web of interpersonal interactions and interrelationships. The baby develops love for his mother within the bounds of an eating situation and whether the enriched meaning of food comes from mother love or the enriched meaning of mother love comes from the satisfactions of eating is a moot point. All through life, enjoyment of life is wrapped up with enjoyment of food. Consider such significant food-involving situations as the family evening dinner, the birthday party, the dating dinner, the Thanksgiving get-together, the wedding breakfast, and the funeral meets. One of the consequences of losses of relatives and friends in old age is a loss of eating companions and, therefore, probably, a reduction in the enjoyment of eating.

The aged can be defined generally as anybody over the age of sixty-five, though if we wish to consider the more feeble, more disabled group, the cutting age is more appropriately seventy-five. The dividing line of sixty-five is customary because it has been set as the legal age for such signaling events as eligibility for Social Security or, in many jobs, compulsory retirement.

The widowed

While most Americans over sixty-five live in their own homes with their own husband or wife, there are many who are residentially isolated. Because, on the average, women live longer than men, there are more residentially isolated old women than old men.[1] Other factors contributing to this unequal sex distribution are the tendency for women to marry older men and the fewer chances for an old widow to find a new husband than for an old widower to find a new wife. However, in part, it is also a question to options. Old widowers remarry more than old widows because there are fewer other alternatives open to them. Old widows can take care of themselves—they are experienced housekeepers; they can move in with a relative (daughter or son, sister, or other); or they can look for a new spouse (and occasionally even find one). Old widowers usually are unprepared to take care of themselves, and most of their contacts with kin have been engineered by their wives so that they are at a loss for communication with children, siblings, and so on. The one arrangement they have been socialized for is with a wife.

Many widows live alone because they like it that way. Lopata studied[9] 301 widows, age fifty or over, in the Chicago area. Half of the sample lived alone, and the proportion increased to a peak of 61 per cent between the ages of sixty-five and sixty-nine.

There is a difference between isolation and desolation.[10] We could describe isolates as those who live alone and like it and desolates as those who live alone but don't like it. Many isolates have lived alone and been "loners" most of their lives.[11] The desolates are the ones who have loved and lost. Their spouses have died; their children live far away; and they haven't adjusted to the loneliness yet—if they ever will. They are the ones we in the helping professions must worry about.

The desolates

How many desolates are there? This cannot be ascertained directly at present. Probably the 4 per cent of those over sixty-five who are in institutions—hospitals, mental hospitals, nursing homes, retirement homes, and so forth—could be so designated.[1] But how many of the 20 per cent of those over sixty-five who live alone should be? Lowenthal compared[11] old-age admissions to the psychiatric ward of the San Francisco County General Hospital with old people living successfully in the community. She found that one of the most significant differences between the two groups was having a confidant: at least one friend who knew whether one were alive and who cared.

Residential isolation could thus be less important than communicative isolation. One could live with other people but if one had no interaction with them, if one's presence were as meaningful to them as a piece of furniture pushed into a corner, one would be more effectively isolated than if one lived alone but talked on the phone daily with a friend on the other side of town, even if one saw that friend rarely face to face.

Within the last ten or fifteen years, a number of intensive research projects on aging have been carried out. One of the earliest and most extensive was the series of Kansas City studies under the direction of the University of Chicago Committee on Human Development.[2,12,13] As the data began accumulating, they pointed to a trend of aging behavior that has been called "disengagement." This refers to a process of withdrawal from social roles and social activity by the aging person that coincides with the simultaneous rejection of the aging person by society. It is not only that society discards its "useless" aged, but that the aged no longer have much use for society.

In the original formulation of this theory, it was assumed that because disengagement was functional, both for the individual and the society, those individuals who disengaged the most would be the happiest. This has not proved to be true. It is the other way around. While there has been repeated replication of the existence of a disengagement process, it has become more and more clear that, in general, those who disengage the least—who remain the most involved in society and the most active, tend to be the most satisfied with their lives and to have the highest morale. To stay alive in the social and psychologic sense, one must act alive.[2]

This rule should not be taken too literally, however. More refined studies, both on the Kansas City data[2] and in California,[14] have shown that in the last analysis, the kind of aging pattern that is the most satisfying to a given individual is a function of his personality. Both studies show more than one type of successful aging, including those who continue to be happily engaged, those who remain engaged but "pushed themselves" because they are afraid to let go, and those who are the contented disengaged, the rocking-chair people who have been looking forward for many years to sitting back and letting others take over and who now feel they have earned their rest.

Food in the aging picture

Part of the goal of any nutrition program for older people, therefore, should be not only to keep them physically alive but also socially and psychologically alive. That means that a good nutrition program for the aged includes more than the proper balance of nourishing food, even nourishing food adapted to the individual's past tastes and prejudices and taboos. It includes at least some opportunity for meaningful social involvement and some opportunity for individual planning and choice of both food and social involvement to suit varying personality types. Recent government-sponsored demonstration projects on the nutrition of the aged have, in fact, been paying particular attention to the multiple facets of the eating experience.[3,15]

At the beginning of this paper, some dilemmas were posed about therapeutic dietetic intervention in old age. Can we now come to any resolution? It seems that the best resolution would lie in considered judgment. Knowing that old people have survived because there was something good in the way they lived and ate, that their eating habits are tied up with what gives meaning and significance to their lives, but that they have changed physically in many cases so that old ways are now no longer so good and also that they have the capacity to change if necessary, the practitioner can balance the pros and cons and come to the wisest decision for each individual.

It could very well be that our potential life span is something we are programmed with at conception.[16,17] Furthermore, the important dietary and other environmental influences on this programming may be those that occur in the beginning of the life span.[3,18] Whether we will live out our potential life span could depend more on our mother's eating habits and her general state of health, and on her care of us in infancy than on anything we ourselves eat in middle or old age. The state of research is still primitive in this respect, but so far as can be judged now, it looks as if dietary intervention in old age is more a maintenance or holding action than a change action. Magic diets, like magic organ transplants, cannot make old men young. Reincarnation is still a religious, not a medical hypothesis.

In conclusion, let me quote from Howell and Loeb[3]: "Many doctors, nurses, social workers, and middle-aged children report that older people, especially those living alone, do not appear to eat enough or to eat a nutritionally balanced diet. However, there is little reported evidence of a high incidence of actual 'clinical' malnutrition among old adults in the United States . . . Better correlation of medical records with dietary history and subjective health reports might help to accumulate needed information on diet and the health status of the aged" (p. 63).

REFERENCES

1. Riley, M., and Foner, A.: Aging and Society. Vol. 1. An Inventory of Research Findings. N. Y.: Russell Sage Foundation, 1968.
2. Neugarten, B.: Middle Age and Aging: A Reader in Social Psychology. Chicago: Univ. of Chicago Press, 1968.
3. Howell, S., and Loeb, M. B.: Nutrition and Aging. A Monograph for Practitioners. The Gerontologist 9: No. 3, Pt. II, 1969.
4. Birren, J. E.: The Psychology of Aging. Englewood Cliffs, N. J.: Prentice-Hall, Inc., 1964.
5. White House Conference on Aging. Fact Sheet, Rev., June 1970.
6. Bromley, D. B.: The Psychology of Human Aging. Baltimore: Penguin Books, 1966.
7. Kuhlen, R.: Age and Intelligence: The Significance of Cultural Change in Longitudinal vs. Cross-sectional Findings. Vita Humana 6: No. 3, 1963.
8. Eisdorfer, C.: Intellectual changes with advancing age: A 10-year follow-up of the Duke sample. Paper presented at a symposium on "Longitudinal Changes with Advancing Age," Amer. Psych. Assn., San Francisco, 1968.
9. Lopata, H.: Living arrangements of American urban widows. Paper presented before Gerontological Society, Toronto, 1970.
10. Lowenthal, M., and Haven, C.: Interaction and Adaptation: Intimacy as a Critical Variable. Amer. Sociol. Rev. 33:20, 1968.
11. Lowenthal, M.: Lives in Distress: The Paths of the Elderly to the Psychiatric Ward. N. Y.: Basic Books, 1964.
12. Cumming, E., and Henry, W.: Growing Old: The Process of Disengagement. N. Y.: Basic Books, 1961.
13. Neugarten, B., Berkowitz, H., and others: Personality in Middle and Late Life: Empirical Studies. N. Y.: Atherton Press, 1964.
14. Riechard, S., Livson, F., and Petersen, P.: Aging and Personality: A Study of Eighty-seven Older Men. N. Y.: John Wiley & Sons, 1962.
15. Pelcovits, J., and Holmes, D.: A nutrition program for Older Americans. Position paper: Nutrition for Older Americans: Demonstration Program Experience. Washington, D.C.: Admin. on Aging, n. d.
16. Comfort, A.: Theories of aging. Paper presented at 8th Intl. Cong. of Gerontology, Washington, D.C., 1969.
17. Strehler, B., ed.: The Biology of Aging. Washington, D.C.: Amer. Inst. of Biol. Sci., 1960.
18. Sherwood, S.: Gerontology and the Sociology of Food and Eating. Aging and Human Development 1:61, 1970.

Recognition and management of grief in elderly patients

EDWIN P. GRAMLICH, M.D.*

Grief is a ubiquitous bodily reaction to emotional injury and loss, not unlike bodily reactions to physical injury. Known throughout the ages as an important cause of illness, it is diffuse in the aged and obscured, if not completely overlooked, in this age of scientific medicine.[1] If it is not truly a disease, as suggested by Engel,[2] it is certainly a state of dis-ease, with organic and physiologic changes. In its uncomplicated form, grief follows a typical and predictable course.[3-7] As with many reactive processes, however, it may follow deviant and atypical courses which are easily confused with other disease processes.[6, 8] The more devious patterns of grief are found in the young and the old.[6] It is stated by Nemiah that melancholia is at the bottom of everything, since nothing lasts and all that is loved or shall be loved must die or be lost.[9] Aging, therefore, subjects individuals to more and more loss. Loved ones are lost, health is lost, cherished goals are unrecognized and lost, cherished occupations and sources of pride and value are lost in the progress of time.[4, 10, 11]

Grief in elderly people has been studied scientifically only on a few occasions[12-15] with contradictory results. Several complete studies of elderly people suggest that grief, as such, may not be a significant event.[15-17] According to the theory of aging proposed by Cummings and Henry, aging people progressively disengage from their environmental attachments and live in an increasingly detached state.[18] It may be, however, that this state is one of a chronic depressive withdrawal and is associated with the continued accumu-

Reproduced from Geriatrics, July, 1968, pp. 87-92.
*Straub Clinic, Honolulu, Hawaii.

lation of losses and overwhelming grief.[1] The recent work of Kastenbaum and Birren supports the general theory that aging is associated with a progressive disengagement from the environment.[15, 16] Their theory proposes that grief in itself is not an essentially important factor, but only one of many stresses applied to the aging individual. Other studies, however, have shown that grief is the precipitating factor in many states of illness and tends to aggravate preexisting organic and psychosomatic disorders.[3, 10, 13, 19-21] The death rate of widows and widowers exceeds that of the population by a significant degree, and it is legendary that many have died of, or at least during, grief.[21]

Definition

To understand grief in the elderly patient, one must have a firm understanding of the general syndrome of grief. The grief process is initiated by awareness of a significant loss. The first reaction to the loss is that of shock and disbelief. This state may be intense and associated with hallucinations and delusions in an effort to deny the loss in fantasy. If the loss is denied by the individual a state of numbness prevails.

Usually the loss can be denied only for a short time. It then becomes painfully obvious to the bereaved person that an extremely important other person has died. This initiates a stage of intense physical distress accompanied by feelings of deep loss and emptiness, associated with intense sadness and sorrow. Physical pain is common, especially headache, muscle and joint pain, and pain and pressure in the neck, chest, and abdomen. It is an all encompassing and disorganizing emotional reaction. It tends to come in waves of pain and distress accompanied by weeping.

This stage usually passes to a more chronic stage of mourning associated with a prolonged feeling of depression and sadness and with periodic memories of the lost person. It is debatable whether typical grief carries with it intense feelings of guilt and hostility. Some authors state that it does, others that it does not.[9, 23] However, it is common to feel intensely hurt and injured. The intensity of the hurt and injury calls for some explanation and meaning on the part of the grieving person. Intense guilt and self-blame often occur and may be of an entirely irrational nature, depending upon the ambivalence of the relationship with the lost person.

Following the guilt, hostility is common. Friends and family members may be confronted with anger and rejection. Efforts to offer comfort may meet with intense hostility. The person views the world as a hostile place, and projects blame to anyone who comes near. As the grieving person continues to do the work of mourning and to cope with the many memories associated with the lost individual, the process slowly subsides over weeks and months until energy is once again available to invest in new people to replace the lost one. This enables the grieving individual to go on and live a life free from the entanglements of the irretrievable past.

Atypical grief

Atypical grief follows one of three general forms: (1) In delayed grief, the loss may be denied for months or years and grief occurs later, inappropriately associated with a reminder of the loss. This frequently occurs on an anniversary of the loss, the individual having experienced no grief prior to that time. (2) Inhibited grief occurs in individuals in whom mourning seems to be subdued; however, it is longer lasting and associated with disturbed behavior or physical symptoms. It is common in young people. (3) Chronic grief is a prolongation and intensification of the normal grief process. It may be associated with states of overactivity without much sense of loss. It may occur in conditions where the grieving individual has identified with the lost person's illness and has developed symptoms similar to those of that illness. These symptoms may persist. It is as though the lost one has become a part of the grieving individual, who attempts to maintain contact with the deceased through illness, or sympathy pain.

Other patterns of chronic grief have to do with chronic isolation and apathy with depression, chronic hostility with paranoid thinking, and lengthy disorganization of preexisting life patterns. Physical symptomatology is a common part of grief, and chronic grief may be manifested by chronic physical symptoms either due to diagnosable psychosomatic conditions or ill-defined symptoms of pain and dysfunction. Parkes[10] lists osteoarthritis, colitis, migraine, asthma, bronchitis, ulcerative colitis, spastic colon, urticaria, and rheumatoid arthritis as disease entities which may be precipitated or aggravated by a loss.

Inhibited grief in the elderly

Typical grief is thought to be uncommon in aged individuals. More often it follows a pattern of inhibited or chronic grief. The most common manifestation of grief in the aged, therefore, is overt somatic pain and distress. Many aspects of grief do not manifest themselves as clearly and are not as well defined as in younger people. It has been shown that elderly patients, who are grieving, frequently present themselves to physicians with physical complaints. They commonly have gastrointestinal symptoms, or joint and muscular pains, or both.

The most important aspect of the diagnostic process is the preceding history of an important loss, perhaps on its anniversary. One should suspect a grief reaction, regardless of the symptomatology, when one sees an individual who has sustained a major loss within the two years prior to the presenting complaints. Most commonly the physician is consulted within six months of the loss and studies have shown that the incidence of office visits is two to three times as great during the six months following a loss as it was during the six months prior to the loss. Since the grieving process is not experienced as intensely on a conscious level in elderly people, it appears that more of the emotional reaction is suppressed and finds an outlet through somatic expression. Most elderly patients actually hurt rather than complain of emotional pain. In my experience, many grieving elderly people also show symptoms of overt emotional and mental disorder, contrary to some of the literature on the subject. This is particularly evident if one takes the time to inquire about the patient's life after the somatic complaints have been investigated. It is my contention that one cannot rule out the grief process in a symptomatic widow unless there is a definite organic disease to explain the symptomatology. Even then, grief may be a strong contributing factor.

Case report An 81-year-old Caucasian widow was seen in psychiatric consultation four months after the death of a favorite but very disappointing son. She complained of abdominal discomfort and lack of appetite. She had been constipated and unable to sleep. She was nervous and frequently tearful. As an occupant of a nursing home, she had been overtly and covertly admonished and accused of being a baby because of her tendency to cry copiously. She had, in effect, been told to "shut up and stop grieving," which increased her grief and denied her an outlet. She expressed much guilt over her son's poor history of accomplishment in life. With encouragement to allow her tears to flow freely, she wept for most of one hour and part of another. The nursing staff was encouraged to assist her in her process of grief and to allow her to weep freely. As soon as this was accomplished, the patient's attitude changed markedly and her symptoms subsided. She developed a more optimistic attitude and began to socialize anew with the members of the nursing home. She resumed her cultural role there as a gossip and on follow-up visits showed only little evidence of residual grief. As the anniversary of her husband's death arrived and of her son's approached, she again experienced her symptoms, but with less intensity.

Treatment

The management of grief in elderly people must be preceded by recognition and understanding of the underlying process. Once the physician is relatively certain that his patient's symptoms are those of grief the course of action is clear, with few exceptions. In the very old patient who is able to deny the loss and live in a state of unreality free from grief, it might be prudent to avoid challenging the denial. However, in the patient with existing symptoms, denial has been unsuccessful. Here, "grief work" must be at least partly done before the patient can be symptom-free to work toward new human relations and some form of partial engagement with the environment. The term "good grief" conveys the concept that grieving is good, necessary, and therapeutic. "Grief work" consists of remembering the lost individual and of working through the pain, guilt, and anger that go with the memories.[9,23] I encourage grieving patients to cry frequently and to freely share their tears with close members of the family, physicians, nurses, and ministers. Paradoxical intention probably operates here, as many people unconsciously do the opposite of what they are told.

I think it important to share guilt, so that it can be forgiven and its irrational aspects rejected. Those who deal with a grieving patient should accept hostility, not react to it with counterhostility. Sharing of guilt feelings often functions to relieve intolerable guilt and may prevent suicide. Also, if it is understood that the patient is simply venting his anger at being hurt by what seems to be an irrational and unjust world, the anger can be accepted as a natural emotional reaction similar to the inflammatory reaction that naturally follows a burn. An angry reaction from a hurt patient should not be taken personally. A tolerant attitude toward it will help the grieving person accept anger and will keep him from directing it inwardly or suppressing it entirely. As this is accomplished, it is important to encourage the process of resocialization and finding new friends to begin, at least, to substitute for the important lost one. Sometimes the grieving process can interfere with current relationships and it is helpful to explain to friends and relatives that the person's hostility or symptom is a part of grief and will subside if they are patient. New living arrangements may have to be made by family members. Tranquilizing and antidepressant drugs can be used, depending on the target symptoms. They help in subduing emotional reactions and allow the individual to take the grief in smaller doses.

Grieving patients should be told that they are in the process of grief and mourning, for many of them do not connect their pain and misery with their loss. They have worked to deny or avoid memory of the loss, with the idea that not thinking about the loss would make the pain go away. Some say it is silly to cry and it does no good to mourn, not realizing that they only fool the mind. The body and emotional self react anyway as the loss is jerked from the very heart of the being and many wounds are opened that must heal. Many interpret their symptoms as a sign of physical disease or mental illness and need to be repeatedly reassured that the symptoms do not represent those dreaded conditions. A few extra minutes of a physician's time and understanding at this point can be exceedingly helpful to a bereaved patient.

Summary

The process of grief in general, and in the aging patient in particular, is outlined. Grief is viewed as a psychosomatic reaction to an extreme environmental stress that every physician should be cognizant of and alert for, especially in the elderly patient in whom it may be hidden behind a facade of somatic complaints. A program of management and treatment is outlined whereby grief can be shortened and prevented from becoming a more chronic and disabling, if not fatal, disease.

REFERENCES

1. Milt, H.: Grief. Trends in Psychiatry. Vol. 3, No. II. West Point, Pa.: Merck Sharp & Dohme, 1966.
2. Engel, G. L.: Is grief a disease? Psychosom. Med. **23**:18, 1961.
3. Kollar, E. J.: Psychological stress. J. nerv. ment. Dis. **132**:382, 1961.
4. Volkan, V.: Normal and pathological grief reactions: A guide of the family physician. Virginia med. Mth. **93**:651, 1966.
5. Parkes, C. M.: Bereavement and mental illness. Part I. A clinical study of the grief of bereaved psychiatric patients. Brit. J. med. Psychol. **38**:1, 1965.
6. Parkes, C. M.: Bereavement and mental illness. Brit. J. med. Psychol. **38**:13, 1965.
7. Lindemann, E.: Symptomatology and management of acute grief. Amer. J. Psychiat. **101**:141, 1944.

8. Engel, G. L.: Grief and grieving. Amer. J. Nursing **64**:93, 1964.

9. Nemiah, J. C.: Foundations of Psychopathology. New York: Oxford: University Press, 1961.

10. Parkes, C. M.: Effects of bereavement on physical and mental health: A study of the medical records of widows. Brit. med. J. **2**:274, 1964.

11. Schmale, A. H., Jr.: Relationship of separation and depression to disease. Psychosom. Med. **20**:259, 1958.

12. Kay, D. W., Roth, M., and Hopkins, B.: Aetiological factors in the causation of affective disorders in old age. J. ment. Sci. **101**:302, 1955.

13. Stern, K., Williams, G. M., and Prados, M.: Grief reactions in later life. Amer. J. Psychiat. **108**:289, 1951.

14. Perlin, S., and Butler, R. N.: Human Aging. U. S. Department of Health, Education and Welfare, National Institute of Mental Health, Bethesda, Md., 1963, p. 159.

15. Birren, J. E., Butler, R. N., Greenhouse, S. W., Sokoloff, L., and Yarrow, M. R.: Human Aging. U. S. Department of Health, Education and Welfare, National Institute of Mental Health, Bethesda, Md., 1963, p. 314.

16. Kastenbaum, R.: New Thoughts on Old Age. New York: Springer Publishing Co., 1964.

17. Simon, A., and Engle, B.: Geriatrics. Amer. J. Psychiat. **120**:671, 1964.

18. Cummings, E., and Henry, W. E.: Growing Old. New York: Basic Books, 1961.

19. Krupt, G. R.: Identification as a defense against loss. Int. J. Psycho-Anal. **46**:303, 1965.

20. Freud, S.: A General Introduction of Psychoanalysis. New York: Washington Square Press, 1960.

21. Young, M., Benjamin, B., and Wallis, C.: The mortality of widowers. Lancet **2**:454, 1963.

22. Kraus, A. S., and Lilienfeld, A. M.: Some epidemiological aspects of the high mortality rate in the young widowed group. J. chron. Dis. **10**:207, 1959.

23. Paul, L.: Crisis intervention. Ment. Hygiene **50**:141, 1966.

Suicide and aging*

H. L. P. RESNIK, M.D.,** and JOEL M. CANTOR, Ph.D.***

The Bureau of Census has estimated that in the year 1970, 20 million persons living in the United States will be aged 65 or over, and because of increasing longevity due to medical advances, there will be 25 million in the year 1985. How many of them will die prematurely by suicide? And, more important, how many will have "died" years before actual physical death?

Suicide causes about 1 per cent of the deaths reported each year; in 1967 that meant about 23,000. The suicide rate has averaged 11 per 100,000 since 1900 for the entire population, but different rates are reported for different groups.[14]

White males over 65 commit suicide three times more often than do white males aged 20-24, and their suicide rate is four times greater than the overall rate for the United States. White females over 65 commit suicide twice as often as white females aged 20-24, although the highest rate occurs earlier, between the ages of 45 and 54. Because at present the recording and reporting of suicide is often incomplete for nonwhites, it is difficult to discern any particular pattern of change for blacks (or nonwhites inclusively). However, the black suicide rate virtually equals the white rate until age 35, when the white rate becomes two to three times higher than the black. Factoring of our urban-rural statistics would probably show that the suicide rate among black adolescents may be higher than among whites living in metropolitan areas. As this young group of nonwhites ages, the reported incidence of suicide among them may be significantly higher.

Marital status seems to influence suicide rates. They are lower for the

Reproduced from Journal of the American Geriatrics Society 18:152-158, February, 1970.
*Presented at the National Conference of Social Workers, New York City, May 27, 1969.
**Chief, Center for Studies of Suicide Prevention, (Room 12A-01), National Institute of Mental Health, 5454 Wisconsin Avenue, Chevy Chase, Maryland 20015.
***Consultant in Program Development, Center for Studies of Suicide Prevention.

111

married and higher for those living alone, through choice or the death of a spouse—a factor not to be ignored in our older population.

Suicide is currently listed among the ten leading causes of death, but more careful and realistic recording might show it to be even more common. Certainly, in most age groups (including the aged), many suicides are concealed in the data for accidents and natural deaths.[15]

Since 1950, there has been a noticeable decline in suicide for those over age 65. The rate for white males aged 65-74 has dropped 26 per cent, and for white females aged 75-84, 25 per cent. There has been a similar decline in England, Norway and Denmark. Farber[2] is of the opinion that the introduction of social security plans reduces suicide potential in the aged by relieving economic distress. We believe this to be only one of a number of variables involved. However, we are concerned here with the increase in the absolute numbers of the aged and the total number of suicides. The aged comprise 9 per cent of the population, yet they contribute 25 per cent of the suicides.

Theoretical considerations

Modern Western psychodynamic thinking about suicide began in the early 1900's with Freud's theory that the unconscious influences man's everyday behavior. He saw two opposing forces at work: an instinct for death, Thanatos, and an instinct for life, Eros. Menninger, writing in 1931 ("Man Against Himself"), broadened the concept of the death instinct and pointed out that man as easily turns his aggression inward as outward, and can use numerous self-destructive opportunities to kill himself. He cited as examples excessive drinking, smoking and auto racing. One might add neglect of one's physical condition, frequent accidents (including automobile accidents) and other risk-taking behavior. Menninger suggested that we think of such behavior as a form of "partial" or "chronic" suicide. He also identified three aspects of the suicide act as manifestations of the death instinct: the wish to kill, to be killed, and to die. When a suicide occurs, the person killed is one who was once loved, then internalized, and then hated. Murder of the hated person results in one's own death. The wish to be killed can be understood as stemming from the guilt associated with the hate, and the person's need to be punished.[3,5] Concepts about death and dying are always relevant when dealing with suicidal persons.

Jung also contributed to our understanding of suicide by suggesting that a person who commits suicide might wish for a rebirth into a more meaningful and spiritual existence. This is a not uncommon wish of older people. Hendin deals with suicide as a dependency conflict, seeing some suicides as acts of retaliation for real or imagined abandonment. "You abandoned me! Now I will abandon you!" Abandonment is very real for many aged people. Horney was one of the first of the psychoanalysts to consider social factors as an influence. Thus suicide could occur when the person was in a state of extreme self-alienation. This can be a realistic reaction to the rejection felt by so many of the aged.[6]

The sociological study of suicide began with the publication of Durkheim's *Le Suicide* in 1897. He had noticed that different suicide rates for various countries and groups remained stable over long periods, and wondered whether such differences might be due to differences in group cohesion. If so, suicide rates might be used as an index of social organization. He also classified suicides into three types: the altruistic (rarely seen with the aged), the egoistic, and the anomic. Maris[8] recently has pointed out that such a classification cannot be considered adequate without the dimension of intrapsychic conflict being correlated with the sociological.

Egoistic suicide occurs in persons living outside of a group, because they are not subject to group inhibitions about suicide and also are deprived of the kind of emotional support available in group membership. Suicide in the aging may be seen as "egoistic" in Durkheim's sense, because the gradual loosening of group ties is a part of the aging process in Western society.

Anomie connotes "normlessness" or absence of group rules regulating conduct. Anomie becomes more of a problem during periods of rapid social change because people become confused as to what is appropriate or proper conduct. Older persons, who often need clearcut guidelines to feel "good" or "safe," may become acutely anxious and disorganized when these guidelines are not present. This factor may well increase suicide in the aged, as our society has not provided identifiable norms for the behavior of older persons.

Indicators of suicidal potential

Some indicators of higher suicide potential, as described by Litman and Farberow,[7] may be applied to aged persons. These variables all contribute toward evaluation of a subject's lethality potential, i.e., the probability for a successful suicide.

Prior suicidal behavior. Various surveys show that 1 in 3 suicide attempters eventually kills himself, and that 1 in 3 completers has a history of prior attempts. Gardner et al.[4] found that, in persons with suicidal histories, suicide occurs nine times more often in those under 55, and eighteen times more often in those over 55. Research findings indicate that aged persons have fewer histories of prior attempts and are also less likely to "cry for help." But when the aged do cry for help, we should heed the communication, as they are much more likely to make an attempt with a more lethal method, and thus be more successful.

Bereavement and loss. Suicide potential is heightened when there has been recent or recurrent loss of loved ones. Moss and Hamilton[10] noted that among the aged, the loss or death of close relatives occurred twice as often for a group of suicide attempters as for a control group. Since loss of relatives and friends as one ages is unavoidable, new relationships must constantly be substituted. As Rachlis[11] has pointed out, the most common losses are of mates, jobs, earnings, physical health and mobility, mental health, life expectancy and status. How many of us can tolerate *one* or more of these insults, especially when we are unable to undo them? Mourning and bereavement become essential problems for the gerontologist, and a comfortable attitude toward them is an essential skill.

Psychiatric disorders. Numerous studies indicate that suicidal behavior occurs more frequently when there is a history of organic brain disease, especially if accompanied by depressive affect. The findings of Gardner et al.[4] in Monroe County, New York show the increasing risk of suicide with psychiatric illness.

Serious physical illness. Serious and chronic health problems causing economic and physical distress may also be an important factor. Frequent exacerbations of chronic illness may increase suicidal potential.

Dorpat et al.[1] studied suicide in patients over the age of 60 and found that 85 per cent of them had an active serious physical illness at the time of death. Apparently, in the aged, the presence of such illness exacerbates the fear of dying, and some of these patients may prefer to precipitate death rather than wait for it passively.

Putting effects in order. Examples of this would be updating a will, changing the beneficiaries of an insurance policy, or giving personal possessions to friends. The victim's behavior not only indicates preparation and planning for death, but might even predate the death by carrying out what usually would be the responsibility of surviving relatives and friends. Putting effects in order, however, may be appropriate and mature. This behavior must be evaluated as one of a constellation of many variables.

Suicidal threats. It is not true, as popularly believed, that those who "talk about it won't do it." Surveys show that high percentages of threateners become attempters, and attempters become completers. In the aged, *all* threats or attempts *must* be taken seriously. The likelihood of a success is many times higher than in other groups. One must be especially careful when the threat is specific about the time, place and method.

Therapeutic intervention

The identification and diagnosis of self-destructive activity is far from even approaching an exact science. Nevertheless, there are some guidelines, as just described. These are based primarily on clinical experience. Current research is aimed at examining these concepts more rigorously.

Mintz[9] has recently outlined the most comprehensive treatment approach.

Treatment is a more serious problem than identification. Patients may be either acutely or chronically suicidal. Whereas crisis intervention on an extremely personal level may suffice for the former, other techniques must be developed for the latter. A depressed aged person is a difficult client. All too often there is pressure for hospital admission, and this may be the best way for a family or a therapist to be rid of ongoing responsibility. We need not remind you that suicidal people kill themselves in hospitals.

Taking action. The first step must be to establish trust. When a suicidal person has given up with regard to his own ability to solve his problems and when the clues to his suicidal intent have been ignored, he may also stop believing that others are interested in helping him. There is more here than simply establishing confidence in a technical ability to help; there must be a demonstration that the patient will be handled with sincerity, warmth and concern. It should not be forgotten that suicide is still taboo to many people.

Once the crisis is understood, it is important that the therapist *act*. Any appropriate realistic step he takes to improve the impasse that overwhelms the victim may lift the feelings of hopelessness and despair. "Taking action" may be no more than a promise of help. It is important also that the therapist be decisive and authoritative because of the confusion and ambivalence felt by the patient. Because the patient's own judgment can no longer be trusted, the therapist must instill confidence that he knows what needs to be done, and will do it. When a life is at stake, the therapist should, if necessary, act *as if* he were omnipotent.

Involving others. The therapist's role as a professional who evaluates the situation and starts a therapeutic and rehabilitative attack on the underlying problem is not enough. He not only must provide the temporary and short-term therapeutic support needed until the emergency subsides, but he must be available for a continued relationship. It is also essential to recruit "significant others" who can help turn the patient back toward life, after they are instructed in the seriousness of the situation, and made responsible for continuing the recovery process. It is bad professional handling to conceal a potential suicide, and it is dangerous for the future of the attempter.

The best therapeutic approach is to have concerned relatives and friends gather to assist and comfort the patient, since this re-establishes the social ties which may have been severed. Too many suicidal and depressed patients are an occupational hazard. The burden should be shared with colleagues, friends and spouse, within professional limits.

In the case of the aged, however, prevention may have to precede intervention immediately before an actual attempt at suicide. Because "normal" aging in Western society is a gradual phasing-out and reduction of activity, the older person can plan and effect an earlier death than necessary, without detection. Numerous self-destructive behaviors and opportunities are available to the older person, e.g., deliberate self-starvation, balking at medically prescribed self-care, hazardous activities, or voluntary seclusion. Any older person living alone, who has lost his self-respect and his group-identity, who has financial difficulty, and who is worried over chronic illness and afraid of tomorrow, is a high risk for suicide.

New techniques must be developed for the case-finding of suicidal persons, especially older ones. Several such techniques include befriending or the "buddy system" of calls or visits, the employment of elderly persons by suicide prevention centers as telephone answerers and as speakers on suicide prevention, and the use of senior-citizen centers for the early identification of suicidal older persons by direct case finding. For instance, try asking the next 100 aged persons, "Have you, in the past, or recently, thought of ending it all?" You won't precipitate an attempt.

There is a growing awareness that the fear of an "old age" death may paradoxically lead an older person to a self-induced, premature death for the purpose of escaping it all. It is also possible that an older person may want to die because he feels that others want him to die.

Here we introduce the concept of self-determined (we have not said suicidal) death for the aged. It is conceivable that as our aged population increases and as our medical and nursing facilities continuously fail to meet the needs, certain selected patients, informed of a fatal illness and prognosis, may be given the privilege and means of ending their own lives. The aged in some cultures and species do this.

The National Center for Studies of Suicide Prevention has allocated a high priority to self-destructive behaviors in the aged and we hope that those who work with this high-risk group will become interested in investigating the problem in depth. There is an unfortunate shortage of skilled mental-health professionals who have a specific interest in treating the dying, the self-destructive and the suicidal, especially when these are old people who may be less useful, less resourceful and less accommodating than younger people.

REFERENCES

1. Dorpat, T. L.; Anderson, W. F., and Ripley, H. S.: The relationship of physical illness to suicide, in Suicidal Behaviors: Diagnosis and Management, ed. by H. L. P. Resnik. Boston; Little, Brown and Co., 1968.
2. Farber, M. L.: Suicide and the welfare state, Ment. Hyg. 49:371-373, 1965.
3. Fenichel, O.: The Psychoanalytic Theory of Neurosis. New York, Norton, 1945.
4. Gardner, E. A.; Bahn, A. K., and Mack, M.: Suicide and psychiatric care in the aging, Arch. Gen. Psychiat. 10:547-553, 1964.
5. Jackson, D. D.: Theories of suicide, in Clues to Suicide, ed. by E. S. Shneidman and N. L. Farberow. New York, McGraw-Hill, 1957.
6. Kastenbaum, R.: Multiple perspectives on a geriatric "death valley," Comm. Ment. Health J. 3:21-29, 1967.
7. Litman, R. E., and Farberow, N. L.: Emergency evaluation of self-destructive potentiality, in The Cry for Help, ed. by N. L. Farberow and E. S. Shneidman. New York, McGraw-Hill, 1961.
8. Maris, R. W.: Social Forces in Urban Suicide. Homewood, Ill., Dorsey Press, 1969.
9. Mintz, R. S.: Psychotherapy of the suicidal patient, in Suicidal Behaviors: Diagnosis and Management, ed. by H. L. P. Resnik. Boston; Little, Brown and Co., 1968.
10. Moss, L. M., and Hamilton, D. M.: Psychotherapy of the suicidal patient, Am. J. Psychiat. 112:814-820, 1956.
11. Rachlis, D.: Suicide and loss adjustment in the aging. Presented at Second Annual Conference, American Association of Suicidology, New York City, March 30, 1969.
12. Walker, D. W.: A study of the relationship between suicide rate and age in the U.S. (1914 to 1964). Program, Annual Meeting, American Statistical Assn., Washington, D.C., 1967.

13. Weiss, J. M. A.: Suicide in the aged, in Suicidal Behaviors: Diagnosis and Management, ed. by H. L. P. Resnik. Boston; Little, Brown and Co., 1968.
14. National Center for Health Statistics: Vital Statistics of the United States. Washington, D.C., Govt. Printing Office.
15. National Center for Health Statistics: Suicide in the United States, 1950-1964. PHS Publication No. 1000, Series 20, No. 5., Washington, D.C., Govt. Printing Office, August 1967.

Brantl + Brown. Readings in gerontology.

We will email you a reminder before this item is due.

Please see http://www.ssl.ox.ac.uk/lending.html
for details on:

- loan policies; these are also displayed on the notice boards and in our library guide.

- how to check when your books are due back.

- how to renew your books, including information on the maximum number of renewals.
  Items may be renewed if not reserved by another reader. Items must be renewed before the library closes on the due date.

- level of fines; fines are charged on overdue books.

Please note that this item may be recalled during Term.